The Diabetes Diet Plan

Quick and Delicious Recipes for Type 2 Diabetes, Prediabetes, and Insulin Resistance

By Connor Thompson

Table of Contents

Contents

Introduction

Dale Evans has rightly said, "Life is not over because you have diabetes. Make the most of what you have, be grateful" (Quotes from diabetics, n.d.).

Diabetes refers to a chronic condition wherein the level of glucose or sugar in the blood becomes very high. If you have diabetes, you may experience symptoms like fatigue, less energy, constant hunger, weight loss, and frequent urination in the initial stages. When the disease develops further, there may be more severe symptoms, such as sores and cuts that take time to heal, yeast infections, foot pain, dark patches on the skin, or numbness in the extremities. If the disease is not managed properly, it can lead to further complications such as cardiovascular disease, kidney damage, nerve damage, and vision loss.

There are various forms of diabetes, but diabetes mellitus type 2 (also referred to as Type 2 diabetes) is the most common. This is a medical condition in which the body's ability to produce insulin is compromised. Insulin is a hormone that is produced by the pancreas and is responsible for regulating the levels of sugar in the blood.

Diabetes has become widely prevalent all over the world. In America, the total annual expenditure on treating this disease exceeds $200 billion.

The foods that people eat and their lifestyle choices play an important role in both preventing and managing diabetes. Research shows that a healthy diet and lifestyle can even help in reversing the condition.

A long-term, large scale study known as the Diabetes Prevention Program (DPP) was taken up with the objective of whether it's possible to prevent diabetes with a healthy lifestyle and diet. One group of people with a risk of getting diabetes mellitus type 2 were given lifestyle and diet intervention. Another group was given a placebo or medication to determine if something could reduce their chances of getting diabetes.

After 3 years, it was observed that the first group's risk of getting diabetes was 58% less compared to the second group, which was given a placebo (Tello, 2018).

The goal of this book is to help you to prevent, manage, and even reverse diabetes using diet and lifestyle interventions. You will be provided with information about the symptoms, which tests can tell whether you have diabetes, and what to do if you are diagnosed with the disease. We will also discuss the reasons for the rise of diabetes, such as overconsumption of processed and sugar-laden food, and the current sedentary lifestyle.

We will discuss what insulin is, what happens when our insulin is constantly elevated, and the problems of insulin resistance.

Topics like what is prediabetes, the risk factors, potential complications, and how to improve and prevent it will be dealt with in the chapter about prediabetes.

In the subsequent chapters, you will get all the information about type 2 diabetes, including the symptoms and complications, causes, risk factors, treatments and medications, as well as common myths.

You will be acquainted with the various ways in which you can deal with the disease, which include intermittent fasting and exercising. You will be informed about the benefits of each, things to keep in mind before exercising, common types of exercise for diabetics, and how to get the most out of your workouts. You will also be provided with a 7-day exercise plan of exercises to include in your daily routine.
After that, you will become familiar with the diabetes diet plan, and which foods to eat and avoid to keep your blood sugar levels under control.

A comprehensive 14-day meal plan has been provided to make eating a simple and easy process. The meals have been designed for people with diabetes and contain diabetes-friendly recipes. Each of the recipes takes only 30 minutes and include a variety of tasty meals for breakfast, lunch, dinner, soups, and snacks.

All the details regarding the nutritional value of each recipe have been specified. A ready-made grocery list has been provided to simplify your task.

If you use the tips given in this book, you can improve and even possibly reverse diabetes.

Now that you know what to expect, we can get started. In the next chapter, we will discuss the reasons for the rise of diabetes and the that insulin plays in the disease.

Chapter 1: The Rise of Diabetes

Diabetes has become very widespread. Over 100 million adults in the US have prediabetes or diabetes.

Here is some statistical information about the disease that can help you to understand the seriousness of the problem.

According to the Centers for Disease Control and Prevention (CDC), in the US, there are more than 30 million people who have diabetes. This is around 10% of the total population.

The ADA has stated that average medical expenditure for people who have diabetes is 2.3 times more than it would have been if the disease did not exist. In 2017, this disease cost the US $327 billion, which includes reduced productivity and direct medical expenses.

In the US, this disease is the 7th main reason for death. It is either the underlying reason or the contributing cause of death.

The World Health Organization has provided information that diabetes was the direct reason for around 1.6 million deaths all over the world in 2016.

The impact of diabetes is widespread, and almost half a billion people's lives are influenced by it. The reason for this alarming situation can be traced back to unhealthy food and lifestyle choices.

In America, many people do not have a balanced diet. Most are eating too much, too often, and the size of the servings are not in proportion to the needs of their bodies. In fact, people eat snacks, pizzas, and desserts at any time of the day.

There is a wide variety of processed and ready-made foods which are tempting and widely available. But they are not healthy because they contain added sugars and trans fats.

Consuming excessive amounts of added sugars can have a negative impact on a person's health. Too many sweetened beverages and foods in your diet can increase the risk of getting heart disease, cause blood glucose problems, and lead to obesity.

A study was conducted by N. T. Nguyen and others to find the relation between obesity and the occurrence of diabetes. There were 21,205 participants in the survey. The results of the survey showed that "In a nationally representative sample of US adults, the prevalence of diabetes increases with increasing weight classes. Nearly one-fourth of adults with diabetes have poor glycemic control, and nearly half of adult diabetics are considered obese suggesting that weight loss is an important intervention in an effort to reduce the impact of diabetes on the health care system" (Nguyen, 2010).

Besides erratic food habits, the lifestyle of Americans is not conducive to their overall well-being. Many people lead sedentary lives and spend long hours sitting at their desks. They don't get enough exercise, are constantly stressed, and fail to get enough sleep. All this leads to higher levels of blood pressure and blood sugar. Moreover, constant nonstop eating leads to elevated insulin over a long duration of time.

Dr Dennis Gage, who is an endocrinologist and works at Park Avenue Endocrinology & Nutrition, New York, says that "Insulin resistance is the major link to Type 2 diabetes. Stress, infection and any environmental factor that causes stress will cause insulin resistance and increase the development of Type 2 diabetes. Type 2 diabetes can be caused by genetic inheritance, but by far, the obesity epidemic has created massive increases in the occurrence of Type 2 diabetes. This is due to the major insulin resistance that is created by obesity" (Caceres, 2017).

Now that we know what one expert thinks, let us see what the connection is between insulin and diabetes.

The Role of Insulin

The hormone produced by your pancreas is known as insulin. It helps your body in using sugar or glucose derived from the carbohydrates present in the foods that you consume for energy. Insulin also enables the body to store this glucose so that it can be used in the future. Besides this, it assists in keeping the levels of blood sugar under control and does not allow them to become very low (hypoglycemia) or very high (hyperglycemia). So, problems can occur when insulin is constantly elevated.

Impact of high levels of insulin:

When the levels of insulin are constantly elevated, the condition is referred to as hyperinsulinemia. Excessive insulin may lead to severe health problems. It has been associated with heart disease, obesity, and cancer. High levels of insulin can make the cells of your body resistant to insulin.

Insulin resistance and increased risk of diabetes:

Excessive body weight, extra fat in the abdominal area, smoking, not getting sufficient exercise, and poor sleep can lead to the development of insulin resistance.

This medical condition occurs when excessive amounts of glucose present in the bloodstream reduce the cells' capacity to absorb blood sugar and use it for energy. The chances of getting diabetes increase due to this because diabetes is a disease which is associated with high and low levels of blood sugar.

According to the estimation of ADA, the American Diabetes Association, almost 50% of the people who have prediabetes and insulin resistance may develop diabetes mellitus type 2 if they do not make any changes in their lifestyle.

Increased risks due to insulin resistance

Insulin resistance increases the chances of high triglycerides, being overweight, and having high levels of blood pressure. Sometimes people may develop acanthosis nigricans or dark patches on the skin.

Effects of resistance to insulin include:

- excessive hunger or thirst
- hunger is not satisfied even after eating
- frequent urination
- feeling more fatigued than usual
- tingling sensation in the feet or hands
- evidence in the blood work
- frequent infections

Tests for insulin resistance: It is usually detected with the help of blood tests. A1C test, fasting blood sugar test, and glucose tolerance tests are used for this purpose.

You can start getting the tests done when you are 40 years old.

The tests are as follows:

A1C test

It is used to measure an individual's average blood glucose levels for the past 2-3 months.

If A1C is less than 5.7%, it is normal.

If A1C is in the range of 5.7% to 6.4%, it indicates prediabetes.

If A1C is 6.5% or more, it indicates diabetes.

However, these numbers may vary by about 0.1% - 0.2% from one lab to the other.

Fasting blood sugar test

This shows an individual's fasting blood sugar level. A person should not eat or drink for a minimum of eight hours before this test is done.

If high levels of sugar are detected, one more test is done after a few days to confirm that the first reading was correct.

If the fasting blood glucose levels are less than 100 mg/dL (milligrams/deciliter), it is normal.

If the levels are in the range of 100 mg/dL - 125 mg/dL, this indicates prediabetes.

If the levels are 126mg/dL or more, this indicates diabetes.

These numbers may vary by 3mg/dL from one lab to another.

Test for glucose tolerance

In this test, the blood sugar level of the individual is determined before the test begins. Then the person is given a sugary drink. After two hours, the person's blood sugar level is examined again.

If the level is below 140mg/dL, it is normal.

If it is in the range of 140mg/dL to 199mg/dL, it indicates prediabetes.

If the blood glucose level is 200mg/dL or more than that it indicates diabetes.

Blood tests

Random blood tests are handy when a person experiences significant symptoms of diabetes. But the ADA does not recommend these tests for determining prediabetes or routine screening for diabetes.

Ways to prevent insulin resistance include:

- Exercising for half an hour, five days a week
- Eating a healthy and balanced diet
- Reducing your weight

We will go over more ways to prevent and fight diabetes later in this book.

David Marrero, who works as the president of education and health care for the ADA, says, "What we know in diabetes prevention, and in prediabetes, is that a very modest amount of weight loss has this huge reduction in risk. You lose 7% of your body weight, you cut your risk [of developing diabetes] by 60%. And, in fact, if you're over 65, it's over 70%."

So, essentially, you need to shed the extra pounds. You can do this by keeping an eye on what you eat and exercising.

In this context, Marrero says, "In your body, what exercise does, is it allows you to bind or uptake insulin more efficiently. You have what they call receptor sites, and the more you exercise, the more active your receptor sites are. And the less you exercise, the less active and responsive they are" (Donovan, J. n.d.).

You can bring your blood sugar levels within the acceptable range by choosing a good lifestyle.

In the next chapter, we will discuss prediabetes, which is also known as glucose intolerance or borderline diabetes. This is a medical condition that occurs prior to the incidence of diabetes mellitus type 2.

You will not only come to know the risk factors, potential complications, and ways to improve and prevent it, but you will also know how to determine whether a person has prediabetes.

Chapter 2: Prediabetes and Type 2 Diabetes

Diabetes is a medical condition that is caused due to elevated levels of glucose or sugar in the blood. There are different types of diabetes, which include prediabetes, type 1 and type 2 diabetes. Let's take a closer look at each below:

Prediabetes

Prediabetes, or borderline diabetes, is a medical condition that occurs prior to the incidence of diabetes mellitus type 2. It is also referred to as glucose intolerance. This implies that the levels of sugar in your blood are more than the normal level. But the levels are not as high as in diabetic patients.

During this phase, the pancreas continues to produce sufficient insulin as a response to the intake of carbohydrates. But insulin is not effective enough to remove sugar from your bloodstream. Therefore, blood sugar remains high, which is a medical condition known as insulin resistance.

Prediabetes is widely prevalent. In 2015, more than 84 million people in America who were 18 years or older had prediabetes. So, you can guess that 1 out of 3 Americans suffered from this condition.

If you have prediabetes, it does not imply that you will develop diabetes. Actually, it gives a warning for the future. Those who have borderline diabetes have a 5-15 times higher chance of proceeding to the next stage of T2D than those who have normal sugar levels.

So, you must take some action in this phase and make healthy changes in your diet and lifestyle.

Usually, no symptoms are visible during this phase, and only 10% of people know that they have prediabetes.

Risk Factors

The factors that can increase the likelihood of the occurrence of prediabetes include:

- Being obese or overweight
- Having a closely related person with diabetes mellitus type 2
- Having high cholesterol
- Being inactive
- Delivering a baby whose weight is over 9 pounds
- Having high blood pressure

How to Know Whether a Person Has Prediabetes

Borderline diabetes does not give any indications and exists silently. Therefore, if you want to know for sure, it is essential to get regular medical checkups done. You can talk with your healthcare provider who will perform an OGTT, oral glucose tolerance test or HbA1c, hemoglobin A1c test.

The hemoglobin A1c test shows the patterns of a person's blood sugar in the previous 2-3 months. It is better than the oral glucose tolerance test because it gives a more comprehensive picture. If the HbA1c level is 5.7-6.4, it indicates borderline diabetes.

Potential Complications

If the high levels of blood sugar are not treated, they can lead to other health complications. You may become vulnerable to various chronic health problems. For instance, uncontrolled diabetes may lead to:

- Cardiovascular disease
- Kidney damage
- Nerve damage

- Vision loss

Moreover, the high levels of insulin that occur due to insulin resistance cause further problems such as heart disease, obesity, and cancer.

Ways to Improve and Prevent Diabetes

The Diabetes Prevention Program, a multicenter research, studied how changes in lifestyle may prevent diabetes. Their findings offer hope for those who have a risk of getting diabetes. In the course of 3 years, those who participated in the study were able to reduce the chances of developing the disease by 58% with moderate exercise and weight loss (Schaeffer, 2018).

This shows that exercise and healthy food play an important role in preventing the disease.

You can take better care of yourself by making simple lifestyle and dietary changes like:

- **Eat healthier:** Include complex carbohydrates and whole foods in your diet such as starchy vegetables, grains, and beans. Cut out simple sugars which raise blood glucose levels and do not provide wholesome nutrition. We will be providing you with a variety of diabetes-friendly recipes later on this book.

  In addition, you can seek the help of a dietitian to plan your meals or refer to the guidelines given by the American Diabetes Association.

- **Exercise:** Make it a point to exercise for at least 150 minutes every week. You can take up any activity that you like; even walking is a good option. You'll be provided with a 7-day exercise plan later on.

- **Lose weight:** You can accomplish this goal by eating healthy food and doing regular exercise.

All this helps to prevent diabetes and avoid potential complications that may occur due to uncontrolled diabetes.

Regarding prediabetes, Dr Kristen Arthur says, "It can be reversed, and you can stop the progression to diabetes" (Schaeffer, 2018).

In the next section, we will look at the difference between type 1 and type 2 diabetes. We will look at the symptoms and complications, causes and risk factors, treatment and medications, and how to manage the disease.

Type 2 Diabetes

As mentioned, diabetes refers to a chronic condition wherein the level of glucose or sugar in the blood becomes very high. Insulin is a hormone that helps to transfer glucose from the blood to the cells where it is utilized for energy.

If you have type 2 diabetes, which is also referred to as diabetes mellitus type 2 or T2D, the cells of your body fail to respond properly to insulin. After a certain stage, your body may even stop producing sufficient insulin.

If T2D is not controlled, there may be high levels of chronic glucose which can cause many symptoms and serious complications like kidney damage, vision loss, cardiovascular disease, and nerve damage.

Difference Between Type 1 and Type 2 Diabetes

Diabetes can manifest as a few different types depending on the causes and nature of the disease. The main types include type 1 and type 2 diabetes.

Type 1 Diabetes

Type 1 diabetes was earlier known as juvenile-onset diabetes. It is also referred to as insulin-dependent diabetes, often starts in childhood, and can be caused due to genetic reasons. Compared to type 2, type 1 diabetes is much less common. It is actually a kind of autoimmune condition wherein the antibodies attack the pancreas. Therefore, the pancreas is damaged and does not make insulin.

Type 2 Diabetes

This type of diabetes is very common and is mild compared to type 1 diabetes. Earlier it was known as adult-onset diabetes and is also referred to as non-insulin-dependent diabetes. In this type of diabetes, a person's pancreas produces some amount of insulin, but it is not sufficient to meet the needs of the body, or the body is resistant to insulin.

Symptoms and Complications

In this disease, the body is unable to use insulin effectively to transfer glucose to the cells. Therefore, it has to depend on other sources of energy in its organs, tissues, and muscles. This chain reaction can lead to various symptoms.

T2D may develop slowly and may show very mild symptoms at the beginning, which can easily be dismissed. The initial symptoms include:

- Fatigue
- Less energy
- Constant hunger
- Weight loss
- Frequent urination
- Excessive thirst
- Itchy skin
- Dry mouth
- Blurry vision

When the disease develops further, there are more severe symptoms such as:

- Sores and cuts that take a lot of time to heal
- Yeast infections
- Foot pain
- Acanthosis nigricans or dark patch on the skin
- Neuropathy or numbness in the extremities

Complications

If diabetes is not managed properly, it can lead to several complications, such as:

- Digestive issues like constipation, diarrhea, and vomiting.
- Poor circulation of blood to your feet. This makes it difficult to heal cuts and infections in the feet. It can even cause gangrene and lead to amputation.
- Hearing may be impaired.
- Deterioration of vision, cataracts, and glaucoma.
- Cardiovascular diseases like angina, stroke, heart attack, and high levels of blood pressure.
- Hypoglycemia may occur when the blood sugar levels are low. Its symptoms include difficulty in speaking, shakiness, and dizziness. In order to rectify the problem, you can take some fruit juice, hard candy, or a soft drink (Pietrangelo, 2019).
- Hyperglycemia may happen when the levels of blood sugar are high. The symptoms of this disorder include increased thirst and frequent urination. Exercising may help to bring down the sugar levels.
- Pregnancy, labor, as well as delivery, can become complicated if a person has diabetes. It can cause harm to the developing organs of the baby. It can also make the baby gain excessive weight put the baby at a greater risk of getting diabetes in the future.

Causes

Your pancreas produces and releases insulin when you have food. When you suffer from T2D, your body develops insulin resistance and does not use the hormone properly. So, your pancreas is forced to make a greater effort to produce insulin.

In the long run, this may damage the cells in the pancreas. Ultimately, the pancreas may stop producing insulin. As a result, glucose gets accumulated in the bloodstream, and the cells of the body do not get enough energy.

Doctors are not sure about what triggers these events. It could be because of cell signaling or cell dysfunction within the pancreas. It can also be because the liver makes excessive amounts of glucose. Otherwise, there could be a genetic reason for developing diabetes mellitus type 2.

Genetic predisposition is definitely connected to obesity. We already know that being overweight increases the likelihood of developing insulin resistance as well as diabetes. An environmental factor could also act as a trigger. Environmental factors include polluted water, air, soil, stress, lack of access to healthy food and vitamin D, and exposure to enteroviruses.

As you can see, a number of factors can increase the chances of the occurrence of the disease.

Risk Factors

The risk factors that are not in your control include:

- If your parent or sibling has diabetes mellitus type 2, you have a greater risk of getting it too.
- Although you can get the disease at any time irrespective of your age, there are more chances of its occurrence after the age of 45.
- Women with PCOS or polycystic ovarian syndrome have a higher chance of getting it.
- People belonging to certain races such as African Americans, Pacific Islanders, Hispanic-Americans, Native Americans, and Asian-Americans are at a greater risk compared to Caucasians.

However, there are a number of factors that are within your control:

- If you are overweight, there are more fatty tissues in the body due to which the cells develop a resistance to insulin. There are more chances for the occurrence of the disease if there is excessive fat in your abdominal area than if there is too much fat in the thighs and hips.

- You are at greater risk if you lead a sedentary life. If you exercise regularly, glucose is used up, and there is an improvement in the response of cells to insulin.
- If you consume too much junk food or eat excessive amounts of food, your blood sugar levels can shoot up drastically.

Besides this, there is a greater risk of getting diabetes if you have had prediabetes or gestational diabetes which are two conditions that occur due to high levels of blood sugar.

Treatments and Medications

If you have T2Dm, you can manage it effectively with the guidance of your doctor. You will have to check the blood sugar levels at certain intervals and maintain them within a particular range. There are a variety of tests that are done to determine the blood glucose levels, which have been explained in chapter one. Not everyone with T2D has to take insulin. Only if your pancreas fails to produce enough insulin will your doctor ask you to do so. Besides this, you can take other medications that your doctor may prescribe.

As we have seen, making changes in your lifestyle may be sufficient to keep T2D under control. Otherwise, you can make use of various helpful medications such as:

- Metformin: This is a preferred medication in most cases of diabetes mellitus type 2. It lowers the blood sugar levels and improves your body's response to insulin.
- Sulfonylureas: These are taken orally and help the body to produce more insulin.
- Meglitinides: These medications act very fast and have to be taken for a short duration. They stimulate the pancreas to provide larger amounts of insulin.
- Thiazolidinediones: They make the body more responsive to insulin.
- Sodium-glucose cotransporter-2 (SGLT2) inhibitors: They help to prevent the reabsorption of glucose by the kidneys and allow it to go out with the urine.
- Glucagon-like peptide-1 (GLP-1) receptor agonists: They slow down the digestion process and bring about an improvement in blood sugar levels.
- Dipeptidyl peptidase-4 inhibitors: They are mild medications that are helpful in reducing blood sugar levels.

If you have some issues regarding cholesterol and blood pressure, you may require some medication for them, too.

You may require insulin therapy in case your body is unable to produce a sufficient amount. You may be given an insulin injection at night, and its effect lasts for a longer time. Otherwise, you may be asked to take several injections during the day.

Keep in mind the medications mentioned may have some side effects. Therefore, you may have to spend some time to find the most suitable medication(s) and treatments for you. As always, speak with your doctor to create a customized treatment plan for your needs.

Managing the Disease

Teamwork between you and your doctor is needed for managing diabetes mellitus type 2. You have to take the medication according to the doctor's instructions and cooperate with them when they want to do the tests. Regular blood tests will show the levels of blood sugar and let you know how well you are able to manage the disease. Diabetes increases the chances of getting cardiovascular disease, so your physician will monitor your cholesterol and blood pressure levels as well.

In addition, you may need some additional tests such as cardiac stress tests or electrocardiogram if there are any indications of a heart problem.

Here are some extra tips to keep to help you manage T2D:

- Eat at set intervals.
- Eat only until you feel full.
- Include healthy carbs and foods that have more fiber in your meals. Eating whole grains, vegetables, and fruits will help in keeping the sugar levels steady. You can refer to chapters four and five to learn about the foods that you should eat and the ones that you must avoid.
- Do not put on any extra weight and be sure to take care of your heart health. That means you should eat only minimal amounts of animal fats, sweets, and refined carbohydrates.

- Do some aerobic activity for 30 minutes every day. This will keep the heart healthy and also control blood sugar. You can have a look at the 7-day exercise plan that has been included in chapter three for more details.
- Take your medication correctly.
- Have your own monitoring system at home. You can use it to test the blood sugar levels on your own on the days when you are not visiting the doctor. You can ask the doctor how often the levels should be tested and what should be the target range.

Lastly, it's a good idea to include your family members in the task of managing the disease. You can educate them about the various symptoms and what to watch out for so they will know what to do in case there is an emergency.

Now that we have a better understanding of type 2 diabetes, the next chapter will show how you can improve your condition or even get rid of the symptoms by adopting a healthy diet and lifestyle.

Chapter 3: Ways to Deal with the Disease

Believe or not, diabetes can be treated and even reversed by changing your eating habits and lifestyle. Medical research done for 20 years has proven that this is true.

A long-term, large scale study known as the Diabetes Prevention Program (DPP) was taken up with the objective of finding out if it is possible to prevent diabetes with a healthy lifestyle and diet.

One group of people who had a risk of getting diabetes mellitus type 2 were given a lifestyle and diet intervention for 24 weeks by the DPP researchers. The aim of the comprehensive lifestyle and diet intervention was to change the daily habits of the participants.

There were lifestyle coaches who interacted with the participants and supervised the sessions meant for physical activities. Sixteen classes were held to teach about basic nutrition as well as behavioral strategies to lose weight. Suitable clinical support was also provided to reinforce individualized plans.

Another group was given a placebo or medication to determine if something could reduce their chances of getting diabetes.

After 3 years, it was seen that the lifestyle and diet intervention was very successful, and the first group's risk of getting diabetes was 58% less than the second group, which was given a placebo.

Participants who were 60 years old or more than showed a better response. They had 71% lesser risk of getting diabetes.

What's more surprising is that these differences lasted for many years. After a period of 10 years, the first group had a 34% lower risk of diabetes than the second group.

Nearly half of the people who participated in the study represented ethnic and racial minorities. All men and women irrespective of their ethnicity showed similar results.

So, as you can see, exercise, weight loss, and diet can not only prevent diabetes but also bring down the blood sugar levels of people who have prediabetes or type 2 diabetes as well (Tello, 2018).

Now take a closer look at one way you can improve your diet and health: intermittent fasting.

Intermittent Fasting

Some research shows that intermittent fasting may be beneficial to help treat or even improve diabetes. Intermittent fasting refers to an eating pattern which comprises cycles of eating with periods of fasting. During the fasting periods, you are not allowed to eat any food — the most common types of intermittent fasting time-restricted eating, alternate-day fasting, and modified fasting.

The most popular type of time-restricted eating is 16:8 fast. This involves fasting for 16 hours a day and eating the other 8 hours. For example, if you limit your eating period from 10 pm to 6 pm and fast from 6 pm to 10 am the next morning, this would be considered a 16:8 fast.

Alternate day fasting involves alternating between days where you eat nothing and days where you eat regularly. The Eat-Stop-Eat method is the most common, which involves fasting for 24 hours once or twice each week.

Lastly, modified fasting (or the 5:2 diet), involves restricting your calories to 25% for two days out of the week. For instance, if your normal daily calorie intake is 2,000 calories, you should limit yourself to a maximum of 500 calories on those two fasting days.

Intermittent fasting offers a wide variety of benefits which include:

- Weight loss

- Improved blood pressure

- Insulin improvement

- Lower blood sugar levels

- Increased metabolism

What Research says about Intermittent Fasting and Diabetes

The BMJ Case Reports journal published an observational study that was done in Canada. In this, the researchers made use of intermittent fasting to decrease diabetic symptoms in patients.

Three men between the ages of 40–67 participated in the study. They were taking drugs as well as insulin on a daily basis to deal with the disease. All of them had high levels of cholesterol and blood pressure.

They attended seminars prior to the study and got all the information about the development, the effects, and the management of diabetes.

After that, two men were asked to abstain from eating food for a period of 24 hours on alternate days. The third person fasted for a period of 3 days every week.

During the days of fasting, they could drink beverages that had low calories such as tea, coffee, and water. Besides this, they could have low-calorie meals in the evenings.

The experiment lasted for ten months; after which the researchers measured their blood glucose and weight.

The results showed significant improvements in men's' health, such as:

- Weight loss

- Lower blood sugar levels

- They could stop the insulin usage after one month when they started the experiment; one person could stop it after five days

- Two of the participants were able to give up all the diabetic drugs. The third participant who was taking four drugs could stop taking 3 of them

So, the researchers concluded that the method of intermittent fasting could be helpful for people who have diabetes. However, the study had only three participants, and more research is needed.

According to the researchers, "This present case series showed that 24-hour fasting regimens can significantly reverse or eliminate the need for diabetic medication" (Townley, 2018).

Another study published in the World Journal of Diabetes, in 2017 and had 10 participants. They were obese, had diabetes, and were taking metformin. The study was done in 3 phases, namely baseline for two weeks, intervention for two weeks, and follow up for two weeks. It showed that it is safe for diabetic people to take up intermittent daily fasting for a short term to improve body weight and fasting glucose.

Finally, a study conducted by M. Mafauzy and others was published in the Medical Journal of Malaysia in 1990. It had 22 participants. It showed that fasting was safe for patients who were taking oral hypoglycemic agents and could help in reducing weight and controlling diabetes.

Although this research is promising, more still has to be done to determine the safety and effectiveness that fasting has on diabetes. If you considering intermittent fasting for any period of time, be sure to talk to your doctor first.

The Role of Exercise

As mentioned, exercising is very beneficial for people with diabetes. Benefits of exercise include:

- Lowers the blood pressure

- Increases the levels of HDL or good cholesterol

- Helps in controlling weight

- Makes the bones stronger

- Helps to build strong muscles

- Makes you feel more energetic

- Improves your mood

- Enables you to relax and sleep better

- Assists in managing stress

Points to remember while exercising:

- Consult your doctor before starting any exercise program

- Always keep some healthy food items with you which you can take if blood sugar drop

- Wear comfortable clothing and shoes

- Keep an eye on the levels of blood pressure

- Start off slowly. If it's been a while since you last exercised, start off with a brisk walk around the block for 20 minutes. Once you are comfortable with this, you can push yourself more, such as by increasing the duration (walk 30 minutes) or intensity (jog or run).

- Aim to exercise 30 minutes each day at least five times a week.

Some common exercises that you can do are:

- Aerobic exercises such as walking, jogging, biking, swimming, dancing, and interval training

- Resistance training which includes weightlifting, and using resistance bands and machines

- Yoga is great for stretching and breathing

- Tai chi in which you do a sequence of actions slowly in a relaxed manner for 30 minutes

In order to get the best results, use the following tips:

- Note down all the activities you enjoy

- Start slowly and gradually increase the time you spend exercising

- Make it a part of your daily routine

- Join a group or class and make it an enjoyable activity

- Listen to your body. If you feel faint or dizzy, stop.

- Test your blood glucose often and be aware of the changes

- Drink sufficient water and keep your body hydrated

- Be realistic while setting your goals

Be sure to choose exercises according to your comfort level and include them in your daily routine. Here is a sample 7-day exercise plan to get you started. However, feel free to add your own exercises according to your needs, interests, and lifestyle.

Day 1

Morning 15 minutes: yoga

Evening 15 minutes: biking

Day 2

Morning 15 minutes: walking

Evening 15 minutes: dancing or jogging

Day 3

Morning 15 minutes: tai chi

Evening 15 minutes: play tennis or basketball

Day 4

Morning 15 minutes: yoga

Evening 15 minutes: jogging

Day 5

Morning 15 minutes: walking

Evening 15 minutes: swimming or hiking

Day 6

Morning 15 minutes: jogging

Evening 15 minutes: hiking on easy terrain

Day 7

Morning 15 minutes: tai chi

Evening 15 minutes: play an outdoor game

In the next chapter, we will discuss what foods to eat and avoid if you have diabetes. We will also show how you can replace unhealthy items with healthier ones.

Chapter 4: Diabetes Diet Plan

Hippocrates, the father of medicine, has rightly said, "Let food be your medicine, and medicine your food."

This same principle applies to diabetes. If you have this condition, this doesn't mean you have to sacrifice all your favorite foods and live a life of deprivation. In fact, you can still choose to eat nutritious foods, balance your meals, and continue to eat foods you love.

Starchy and sugary carbohydrates may raise the levels of blood sugar, so you can include them in the right proportions and plan a balanced diet for yourself.

It's necessary to keep a check on the total quantity of carbohydrates that are consumed in every meal when you have diabetes. The allowable level of carbs is different for each person, as it depends on the needs of their body. This is based on several factors, such as how active you are and what medications, like insulin, you are taking.

You can consult a dietitian who can guide you and recommend the right amount for you on the basis of your needs. However, the general rule postulated by the Academy of Nutrition and Dietetics states that starchy carbohydrates in a single meal should be equal to just one-quarter plate.

In this chapter, we will tell you about the glycemic load and glycemic index, which indicate the influence of particular carbs on the level of blood sugar. Under the topic 'Food Choices', you will get some guidance about choosing the right carbohydrates to help balance your blood sugar levels.

You will also learn about different types of carbohydrates, fats, and protein, and which are recommended for people with diabetes. Lastly, we will show you how to choose your desserts and plan your meal and portion sizes.

Glycemic Load and Glycemic Index

Carbohydrates are the main foods that raise blood sugar. GL (glycemic load) and GI (glycemic index) are two scientific terms that are used for measuring the influence of particular carbs on the level of blood sugar.

The food items that have a lower glycemic index raise the sugar levels moderately. Therefore, they are a better choice for those who have diabetes.

The quantity of fiber, protein, and fat present in a food item or meal determines its glycemic load.

The term glycemic index refers to a standard measurement, while the glycemic load takes into account the portion sizes in real life. For instance, one bowl of green peas has a GI of 68 (per hundred grams) and GL of 16 only. If you take only the GI into consideration, you may think that peas are not suitable for you. But you are likely not going to eat 100g peas at one time. So if you eat a common portion size, you will see that the glycemic load of peas is quite healthy. Besides this, peas are very rich in protein and therefore a good choice. However, there are some limitations to this model.

Limitations of Glycemic Index:

- The exact health advantages of using the glycemic index are not known.
- Eating becomes a complicated affair when you have to refer frequently to glycemic index tables.
- The glycemic index does not measure the healthfulness of food.

Research has shown that if you follow the guidance given by any of the heart-healthy diets, such as the Mediterranean diet, you can reduce the glycemic load and enhance your diet's quality (Segal, Robinson & Smith, 2019).

Food Choices

When choosing foods, you should choose carbohydrates that have plenty of fiber and won't raise the blood sugar levels. For instance, here are some healthier alternatives to common foods:

- White rice better options: Brown rice, wild rice, and riced cauliflower
- White potatoes (inclusive of mashed potatoes and fries) better options: Yams, sweet potatoes, and cauliflower mash
- Regular pasta better options: Spaghetti squash and pasta made with whole wheat
- White bread better options: Bread made with whole grain or whole wheat
- Sugary breakfast cereal better options: Low-sugar and high fiber cereals
- Instant oatmeal better options: Rolled oats and steel-cut oats
- Cornflakes better options: Low-sugar type of bran flakes
- Corn better options: Leafy greens and peas

Types of Carbohydrates

There are two types of carbohydrates, namely complex carbohydrates and simple sugars.

Complex carbohydrates are foods that have low glycemic loads or are included in low-carb diets meant for diabetes type 2. They are in full form and contain extra nutrients like:

- Fiber
- Vitamins
- Some amount of fats and proteins

Carbohydrates influence the levels of blood sugar to a greater extent compared to proteins and fats. Therefore, you should be very careful about the types of carbohydrates you choose to eat. Reduce your intake of refined carbs like white rice, pasta, and bread. Take limited amounts of snack foods, packaged meals, soda, and candy. Opt for complex carbohydrates that have more fiber or slow-release carbohydrates, since these are digested slowly and prevent the body from producing excessive insulin.

Types of Recommended Fats

Fats do not have much influence on the levels of sugar in the blood. However, as they are a part of a meal, they can help to slow the absorption rate of carbs into the body. Moreover, they also have a positive impact on your health. Some health examples include:

- Fats found in animal meats increase the chances of the occurrence of cardiovascular diseases. But dairy, especially fermented dairy products like yogurt, may reduce this risk.
- Fats that are plant-based like olive oil, avocado, seeds, and nuts may be associated with a lower risk of incidence of cardiovascular diseases.
- Fats also provide a sense of satisfaction. They can help in dealing with a tendency to overeat and a craving for carbohydrates. For instance, eating one helping of healthy fat such as avocado with a whole grain slice of bread is more healthful and satisfying than jam and a slice of white bread.

Unhealthy Fats

Artificially made trans fats can wreak havoc on your health. Thus, it's better to use vegetable oils instead. You should avoid commercially packaged snacks, baked goods, and fried food. Stay away from any of the food items in which "partially hydrogenated" types of oil have been used even if the manufacturer claims that it is free from trans fats.

Healthy Fats

Unsaturated fats are the healthiest types of fats. They are derived from plant sources like avocados, nuts, olive oil, and fish. Omega 3 fats are conducive for heart and brain health and help to reduce inflammation. Flax seeds, salmon, and tuna are good sources of this type of fat.

Saturated Fats

Saturated fats are mainly found in dairy, tropical oils, and red meat. You do not have to exclude saturated fats from the diet, but they can be consumed in moderate quantities. According to the American Diabetes Association, a person should derive only up to 10% of their calories per day from saturated fats (Segal, Robinson & Smith, 2019).

Ways to Replace Unhealthy Fats with Healthier Ones:

- You can eat nuts and seeds or put them in your bowl of cereal instead of eating chips and crackers.
- Broil, stir-fry, or bake foods instead of frying them.
- Avoid buying and consuming take out foods, packaged meals, as well as processed meats. This will help you to stay away from saturated fats.
- Instead of red meat, try to include a variety of protein-rich vegetarian sources, fish, eggs, and skinless chicken in your diet.
- Opt for extra virgin olive oil when making salad dressings, and cooking pasta or vegetables.
- Commercial dressings often contain trans fats and have high calories. You can make your own healthy dressings with sesame oil, olive oil, or flaxseed oil
- Use avocados to make guacamole or add them to salads and sandwiches. They contain plenty of healthy fats and make you feel full and satisfied after a meal.
- Consume moderate quantities of dairy products.

Kinds of Proteins to be Taken

Proteins have very little impact on the presence of sugar in the blood. They are a source of slow and steady energy and help to stabilize blood sugar levels. Proteins also provide a feeling of satisfaction after eating and help to keep sugar cravings at bay. Therefore, you should include proteins, especially those that are derived from plants, in your meals or snacks.

You can get proteins from both plant and animal sources; however, animal sources may provide some unhealthy type of saturated fats.

Suitable Sources of Proteins Include:

- The organic type of dairy products
- Seafood and fish
- Eggs
- Beans
- Legumes

- Peas
- Soy foods and tofu
- Lean meats like turkey and chicken

You should focus on balancing the macronutrients like carbohydrates, fats, and proteins in each meal to keep the levels of sugar stable. You can plan your meals so that you can get 20% to 35% of the day's total calories from fats. The ADA recommends that you should derive just 10% of your daily calories from proteins. However, you should consult a dietitian to know the exact quantity of carbohydrates that you can have on a daily basis (Williams, n.d.). They may recommend that carbohydrates should provide 55% to 65% of your daily calories.

 You must be more careful about the consumption of fiber, fat, and proteins because they are responsible for slowing down the absorption of carbohydrates. This, in turn, slows down and reduces the production of insulin. Consequently, glucose is steadily transported from the blood to the various tissues.

Making Smart Sweet Choices

Don't think you have to give up your favorite sweets just because you have diabetes. The good news is that you can continue to enjoy small servings of sweet dishes at certain intervals. The main thing is that it should be done in moderation. Here are things to keep in mind:

- Gradually decrease your craving for sweets: reduce the amount of sugar that you eat gradually over time. This will enable you to develop a taste for food items that contain less sugar.
- Cut out the carbs: if you are planning to have a dessert, cut out the pasta, rice, or bread item from that meal. When you eat sweets, your body gets carbohydrates so you should eliminate the other foods that are rich in carbs from that meal.
- Add healthy fats: fats slow down the digestion, meaning that the sugar levels do not rise as quickly. However, you should be careful while doing this and add healthy fats like ricotta cheese, peanut butter, nuts, or yoghurt.

- Eat sweets along with the meal instead of eating them as a separate snack: if you eat sweets separately, they can make the blood sugar rise quickly. However, when they are eaten with other healthy food items, blood sugar does not rise as swiftly.
- Enjoy each and every bite: do not eat a huge chunk of cake or a bag full of cookies without being conscious of what you are doing. You should eat slowly and relish the flavors. Enjoy the treat thoroughly. This will give you more satisfaction and prevent you from overeating.
- Reduce your intake of juice, soda, and soft drinks: for every 12 oz of a sweetened drink consumed per day, the chances for getting diabetes increase by nearly 15%. Instead, drink a lime or lemon drink with sparkling water. You should also reduce the number of sweeteners and creamers that you use with coffee and tea.
- Do not make the mistake of replacing saturated fats with sugar: sometimes people replace whole milk products with refined carbohydrates thinking that it is a healthier choice. However, when fats are substituted with items that contain added sugars (even if the items are low-fat), they are still unhealthy.
- Sweeten food items yourself: for example, you can buy unsweetened plain yoghurt, iced tea, and unflavored oatmeal. Then you can add fruits or sweeteners according to your choice. This allows you to add less sugar compared to those found in the supermarket.
- Avoid processed foods: try to prepare meals on your own instead of buying frozen dinners, canned soups, and packaged meals that often have hidden sugar.
- Read the labels: Read the ingredients and nutrition facts on food items and choose those with low sugar content. Opt for fresh and frozen items rather than choosing canned goods. Pay special attention to the quantity of sugar present in sugary drinks and cereals.
- Decrease the quantity of sugar by ⅓ or ¼ while following a general recipe: you can use vanilla extract, mint, cinnamon, or nutmeg to boost the sweetness.
- Find healthy alternatives to satisfy your sweet tooth: you can opt for a tasty creamy smoothie made with frozen bananas instead of ice cream, or have some dark chocolate instead of milk chocolate.
- Reduce serving size: you can have half of the usual serving and add fruit for the remaining half instead.

To better manage your diabetes, you should balance the low-GI and high-GI food items. The foods that have a high-GI increase the levels of sugar in the blood more than the ones that have a low-GI.

While choosing foods with a high GI, limit the portion sizes. Pairing these food items with healthy fat or protein will reduce their influence on blood glucose and make you feel satiated for a longer time.

Foods with a high-GI are:

- White rice, pasta, bread, potatoes

- Puffed rice

- Pumpkin

- Pineapple

- Melons

- Popcorn

There should be a balance between the following:

Food items that are rich in carbohydrates: Carbs are important components of meals. You can limit their intake or pair them with healthy sources of fats and protein. For example, you can eat eggs and rolled oats with nuts and seeds for breakfast. Or have brown rice with beans, legumes, peas, or skinless chicken cooked in olive oil for a meal.

Fruits that have high-GI: Pineapples and melons have a high GI so they can raise the blood sugar levels. However, many other fruits have a low GI such as cherries, plums, apples, grapefruit, pears, and oranges.

Trans and saturated fats: Unhealthy fats may make things worse for a diabetic person. Many processed and fried foods, including chips, baked goods, and fries, contain these kinds of fats.

Sweetened drinks: Energy drinks, shakes, and sodas contain lots of sugar and can spike your insulin levels.

Refined sugar: Refined sugar is made by processing sugar to make it white and fine. Due to this, it loses all nutrients. This type of sugar is broken down rapidly by the body. As a result, the blood glucose levels shoot up. As refined sugar gets digested very quickly, you do not feel full even after eating a lot of it. So, you should eat fewer biscuits, cakes, and sweets that contain refined sugar.

The American Heart Association recommends that women should not take more than six teaspoons or 24 g, and men should limit their intake to 9 teaspoons or 36 g per day of added sugars. Natural sugars present in plain milk and fruits are not included in this.

Salted foods: Foods which contain a lot of salt can increase your blood pressure. Sometimes sodium may be written on the food label instead of salt.

The ADA recommends that people, including diabetics, should take less than 2300 mg per day of sodium.

Alcohol: You can consume limited amounts of alcohol. Men and women can take two and one drink per day, respectively. Keep in mind, if you are using insulin secretagogue therapy or insulin, there is a risk of getting hypoglycemia connected to alcohol intake. As always, be sure to talk to your doctor to see if it's safe for you to take alcohol.

In the next chapter, you will learn which foods to eat if you have diabetes.

Chapter 5: Most Suitable Foods for Diabetes

In this chapter, we will go over some of the best foods to have if you have diabetes. We will also discuss their benefits and how they can help you to improve your health.

Fatty Fish

Fatty fish is considered to be the healthiest food around. Sardines, salmon, herring, mackerel, and anchovies are excellent sources of omega-3 fats EPA and DHA, which are extremely beneficial for the heart. If there is inflammation within the body, it can damage the blood vessels and potentially cause strokes and heart disease. The fatty acids help to reduce inflammation and prevent these problems. Moreover, they are beneficial for heart health as they decrease triglycerides, lower blood pressure to a certain extent, and reduce blood clotting.

Consuming enough healthy fats is important for people with diabetes as they have a greater risk of getting a stroke and heart disease.

A study conducted by J. Zhang and others was published in the British Journal of Nutrition in 2012. It showed there was a significant reduction in inflammatory markers and triglycerides in older women and men who ate fatty fish 5 to 7 days every week for a period of 8 weeks (Spritzler, 2017).

Leafy Greens

Kale, spinach, and other leafy green vegetables provide numerous essential minerals and vitamins such as vitamin C.

One study showed that increasing the intake of vitamin C reduces fasting blood glucose levels and inflammatory markers for people who have high levels of blood pressure or diabetes mellitus type 2 (Spritzler, 2017).

Cinnamon

Cinnamon not only tastes great, but it's also great for your health. Hemoglobin A1c refers to glycated hemoglobin or hemoglobin with attached glucose. You already know that hemoglobin A1c is a test which is done to determine an individual's average blood sugar level in the past 2-3 months. It measures glycated hemoglobin's percentage in the individual's blood. If it is high, the person suffers from the symptoms of diabetes.

A study showed that the hemoglobin A1c was reduced by two times in diabetic patients who ate cinnamon for a period of 90 days compared to the others who were given only standard care (Spritzler, 2017).

Besides this, R.W. Allen and others did an analysis of about ten studies. It was published in the Annals of Family Medicine in 2013 and showed that cinnamon could also lower the levels of triglyceride and cholesterol.

However, some varieties of cinnamon should be taken in limited quantities, such as cassia cinnamon.

Eggs

Eggs are delicious and filling. Moreover, eggs are great sources of zeaxanthin and lutein, antioxidants which provide protection to the eyes. Eating eggs on a regular basis can also reduces the risk of heart disease.

A study in which diabetic people ate two eggs every day while following a diet that was high in protein showed improvements in the levels of blood sugar and cholesterol (Spritzler, 2017).

Generally, it's better to consume whole eggs as there are a lot of nutrients in both the yolks and whites.

Chia Seeds

Chia seeds have plenty of fiber and less digestible carbs. One ounce or 28 g of these seeds contain 12 g of carbs (out of which 11 g are fiber), so they won't raise blood glucose levels.

Fiber slows down the movement of food through the gut as well as its absorption. It is filling so it can help to reduce the number of calories consumed.

Chia seeds can also help in reducing inflammatory markers and blood pressure.

Turmeric

Turmeric contains curcumin which can lower blood sugar levels and reduce inflammation. It is conducive for kidney health, which is significant for people with diabetes because diabetes is an important cause for kidney disease.

However, curcumin may not be absorbed properly until it is accompanied by piperine. This is an alkaloid that is present in black pepper and is responsible for its pungency.

Greek Yogurt

Greek yogurt tastes great and contains probiotics, which reduce the risk of heart disease. Studies have shown that it may help in weight management and improve the body composition of diabetic people (Spritzler, 2017).

It is best to buy the plain, full fat, organic, or the grass-fed varieties of Greek yogurt. Some of the good quality brands that you can choose to buy are Kalona Super Natural Organic, Maple Hill Creamery, Redwood Hill Farms, and Wallaby Organic.

Nuts

Almonds, walnuts, pistachios, cashews, hazelnuts, pecans, and macadamia nuts are very healthy for diabetic people. They contain fewer digestible carbohydrates and help to reduce the levels of insulin, blood sugar, and LDL cholesterol.

A study conducted by L.C. Tapsell and others was published in the European Journal of Clinical Nutrition in 2009. It showed that diabetic people who ate 30g of walnuts on a regular basis for a year had reduced insulin levels, lost weight, and their body composition improved (Spritzler, 2017).

Broccoli

This superfood is low-carb and low-calorie and offers plenty of nutrients. It is full of healthy compounds that provide protection against several diseases.

Studies have shown that consuming broccoli can help in protecting cells from free radicals. Free radicals are produced in the course of metabolism and help in lowering the levels of insulin (Spritzler, 2017).

Extra-Virgin Olive Oil

Extra virgin olive oil can be added to just about any meal, including salads and bread. It's beneficial for the heart since it has oleic acid that is monounsaturated fat which improves HDL and triglycerides. In addition, it may increase GLP-1, the hormone that makes you feel full.

In an analysis of about 32 studies looking at different kinds of fats, it was seen that only olive oil reduced the risk of heart disease (Spritzler, 2017).

Flaxseeds

Flaxseeds can help in reducing inflammation, decreasing blood glucose levels, lowering the risk of heart disease, and improving insulin sensitivity.

A study showed that after a period of 12 weeks, there was a big improvement in the hemoglobin A1c of diabetic people who ate flaxseed lignans regularly (Spritzler, 2017).

Another study showed that there is a possibility of reducing the medication for the prevention of blood clots and decreasing the chances of strokes with the help of flaxseeds (Spritzler, 2017).

Apple Cider Vinegar

Apple cider vinegar is one of my favorite superfoods. Not only can it lower blood glucose levels and improve insulin sensitivity, but it can also make you feel fuller for longer.

A study published by Andrea and Carol in Diabetes Care in 2007 showed that the fasting blood glucose of diabetic patients who had uncontrolled blood sugar levels was reduced by 6% when the patients took a small amount (2 tbsp) of vinegar before going to bed (Spritzler, 2017).

Garlic

Garlic not only adds flavor, but it also adds many health benefits. It helps to reduce blood sugar, LDL cholesterol, blood pressure, and inflammation in diabetic people.

A 12-week study conducted by K. Ried and others was published in Maturitas in 2010. It showed that the blood pressure of subjects with uncontrolled high levels of blood pressure decreased by approximately 10 points when they ate aged garlic regularly (Spritzler, 2017).

Squash

Squash has become one of my favorite vegetables over the years. It makes a great side dish and contains plenty of beneficial antioxidants. A number of winter squashes have a high content of zeaxanthin and lutein which help to protect against macular degeneration and cataracts.

Some studies conducted on animals, in which squash extracts were used, showed that it might be able to bring about a reduction in insulin levels and obesity (Spritzler, 2017).

A study conducted by J.L. Acosta-Patino and others was published in the Journal of Ethnopharmacology in 2001. It showed that the blood glucose levels decreased significantly for people with diabetes who ate the extract of Cucurbita Ficifolia, a winter squash (Spritzler, 2017).

Keep in mind that winter squash contains more carbs compared to the summer varieties. For example, a cup of pumpkin has 9 g of digestible carbohydrates while a cup of zucchini contains just 3 g of digestible carbohydrates.

Shirataki Noodles

These tasty noodles are excellent for weight control and diabetes. They contain a lot of fiber known as glucomannan and helps to satisfy your hunger.

A study conducted by V. Vuksan was published in Diabetes Care in 1999. It showed that glucomannan reduces the risk factors for heart disease in diabetic people and lowers blood glucose levels (Spritzler, 2017).

Whole Grains

Whole grains are better than refined grains as they contain more nutrients. They have plenty of fiber which is helpful for diabetic people because it slows down the digestion process. Blood glucose levels remain stable when the nutrients are absorbed slowly.

Rye, bulgur, brown rice, millet, quinoa, and buckwheat are some good whole grains for people with diabetes.

Beans

Beans have a low GI and are better than other starchy food items for blood glucose regulation. Besides this, they can be helpful in managing the sugar levels because they are complex carbohydrates and get digested slowly.

Kidney beans, navy beans, black beans, pinto beans, and adzuki beans are good choices for people with diabetes.

These beans provide important nutrients like iron, magnesium, and potassium. They are very versatile and can be included in various dishes such as stews, salads, and tortilla wraps.

Walnuts

They contain healthy fatty acids such as alpha-lipoic which are good for the heart. Diabetic people have a greater risk of getting a stroke or heart disease. Therefore, it's essential to include the sources of such fatty acids in the diet. Walnuts also contain important nutrients like protein, iron, vitamin B-6, and magnesium. So, eating a handful (about seven walnuts) every day is good for health.

A study conducted in 2018 showed that consuming walnuts has some connection with a lower occurrence of diabetes (Sissons, 2019).

Citrus Fruits

Research shows that oranges, lemons, grapefruits, and other citrus fruits have antidiabetic effects.

A few researchers are of the opinion that naringin and hesperidin are the bioflavonoid antioxidants which are responsible for orange's antidiabetic effects (Sissons, 2019).

A study conducted by U.J. Jung and others was published in the Journal of Nutrition in 2004. It showed that antioxidant compounds like bioflavonoids might provide protection against diabetes and prevent the occurrence of complication to a certain extent.

Berries

Berries are rich in antioxidants and can help in reducing oxidative stress. Oxidative stress is associated with a number of health issues, including cancer and heart disease.

Studies have shown that diabetic people have chronic oxidative stress. It takes place when there is an imbalance between the free radicals and antioxidants in a person's body (Sissons, 2019).

So, it is good to eat berries such as blackberries, strawberries, blueberries and raspberries if you have diabetes.

Sweet Potatoes

Sweet potatoes are ideal for people with diabetes since they release sugar slowly and won't raise blood sugar levels too much. They also provide fiber, potassium, and vitamins A and C.

The tasty vegetables can be eaten in various ways, including baked, mashed, boiled, or roasted. You can pair them with green leafy veggies, a salad, or any other sources of lean proteins.

In the next chapter, we will discuss the myths associated with diabetes.

Chapter 6: Diabetes Myths

There are a number of myths that are associated with diabetes. Some of these notions are partly true, but many of the ideas are false. For instance, many people think that sugar is the root cause of diabetes and should be given up. Or that carbohydrates are bad so all types of carbohydrates must be eliminated. However, these ideas are false. As we have discussed, our bodies need the proper amounts of protein, fats, carbs, and sugars to keep it fueled. The problem is most people typically consume too many sugars, carbs or fats. Therefore, the most important aspect for your diet is having a well-balanced meal.

Let's take a closer look at some common myths below:

1. You should give up sugar

As we have mentioned, you don't have to give up your favorite desserts if you eat them with healthier food options. Therefore, it's necessary to plan your meals ahead of time and limit your consumption of hidden sugars.

2. You need to reduce your consumption of carbohydrates greatly

This depends on the kind of carbs you eat and the serving size. Instead of eating starchy carbs, you should focus on carbs derived from whole grains. They contain plenty of fiber, get digested slowly, and keep the blood glucose levels balanced.

After fasting for a minimum of eight hours, normal blood glucose levels can be up to 100 mg/dL. The glucose level can be up to 140 mg/dL two hours after eating.

3. A high-protein diet is best

Studies show that if you eat excessive protein, especially protein derived from animal sources, you may develop insulin resistance. As we have discussed, insulin resistance is a common symptom of diabetes (Segal, Robinson & Smith, 2019). Your body needs the right amounts of protein, fats, and carbohydrates to function well. So, you should eat meals which are healthy and balanced.

The ADA recommends that you should derive just 10% of your daily calories from proteins.

Good sources of protein include eggs, seafood and fish, beans, peas, legumes, organic dairy products, tofu, soy foods and lean meats like turkey and chicken.

4. You should avoid potatoes

It's true that potatoes contain a lot of carbohydrates. However, you can still eat them in moderate amounts. You may even eat other foods that are rich in carbs like rice, pasta, and bread in moderation. You can have 15 to 20 g per snack and 45 to 60 g of carbohydrates per meal.

5. Sugar-free and diabetes-friendly food items are better

These food items are just like regular ones but do not provide any special benefits for people with diabetes. Moreover, they are quite expensive. So, it's better to eat healthy and nutritious whole foods instead of the processed sugarless ones.

6. Sugar is the cause of diabetes

The ADA has clarified that a person does not get diabetes just by eating excessive sugar, although sugar can be one of the contributing factors for the disease. The causes of T1D include genetic and autoimmune responses. The causes of T2D include lifestyle, obesity, and age.

However, recent studies have shown that sweetened beverages like fruit punches and sodas have an excess of empty calories, which increase the risk of diabetes. So, the ADA recommends that they should be avoided (McDermott and Gotter, 2016).

7. You should not drink alcohol

If your sugar levels are under control, you can consume moderate amounts of alcohol. According to the Dietary Guidelines for Americans, women can have one alcoholic beverage and men can have two alcoholic beverages per day. One beverage is equal to 5 oz wine, 1.5 oz distilled spirits, or 12 oz beer.

After drinking, you should monitor your blood sugar levels for about 24 hours. Alcohol consumption may cause the levels to drop below normal, prevent the production of glucose by the liver, and interfere with medications.

8. Avoid fruits

None of the fruits are forbidden for people with diabetes. Although some fruits do contain a lot of natural sugars, you can eat them as long as the serving size is small.

For instance, it's safe to eat one serving of fruits like banana, pineapple, mango, and strawberries. This is equal to half a medium-sized banana, three and a quarter cups of cubed pineapple, half a cup of cubed mango, and one and a quarter cup of strawberries.

9. You can eat whatever you like even when you are taking medication

Taking diabetic medication doesn't give you the freedom to eat whatever you want. In order to get the medication's full benefit, it's important to follow your doctor's instructions and eat healthy well-balanced meals.

Now that we have dispelled some common myths, you'll be provided with a grocery list which will come in handy when you follow the diabetes diet plan for the next 14 days.

Chapter 7: Grocery List

This is a grocery list for the recipes included in the 14-day diet plan in this book. It is divided into two sections: The first section contains all the ingredients that you will need for preparing breakfast items and snacks. The second section has an extensive list of all the things you will need for making lunch and dinner recipes. Besides this, you will also find a list of kitchen tools that are required.

Breakfast and Snacks

Butter

- almond butter
- peanut butter

Honey

- 15 oz honey

Seeds and Nuts

- almonds
- pumpkin seeds
- chia seeds
- flaxseed meal

Oats

- 16 oz oats (rolled)

Eggs

- 10 eggs

Meat and Fish

- 2 turkey slices

- 8 bacon slices
- 28 oz salmon (smoked)

Seasonings and Flavors

- 5 spice powder
- cinnamon
- salt
- black pepper
- cumin
- coriander
- fresh rosemary
- vanilla extract
- lemon zest

Fruits

- 6 avocados
- 1 pear
- 1 apple
- 10 oz frozen blueberries
- 8 cherries
- 1 oz pineapple slices (frozen)
- 1 oz mango slices

Vegetables

- 20 oz carrots
- 1 cucumber
- 26 peppers
- 1/2 red onion
- Onion sprouts
- 2 garlic cloves
- 4 celery sticks (4 inches each)
- 6 lemons

Dairy

- cream cheese
- salmon flavored cream cheese
- 16 oz yogurt

Non-Dairy

- 20 oz almond milk (unsweetened)

Oil

- coconut oil
- 2.5 oz olive oil

Others

- almond flour
- baking soda
- tartaric acid
- pumpkin puree
- 12 flour tortillas
- chocolate chips

- 2.25 (15 oz) cans of chickpeas
- shredded coconut

- 1 oz sriracha sauce

- 8 slices pita bread
- 8 bread slices

Lunch and Dinner

Grains

- 2 oz corn (whole kernel)
- 8 oz pearl barley (whole grain)

Beans and Lentils

- kidney beans
- chickpeas
- red lentils
- green lentils (sprouted)

Eggs

- 2 eggs

Fish

- 48 oz Arctic Char (wild salmon, thick fillets are preferable as it is easier to cut them into cubes)
- 4 oz tuna chunks

Meat

- 2 lb turkey
- 28 oz chicken breasts (boneless, skinless)
- 6 oz chicken breast
- 24 oz minced chicken
- 4 slices of bacon
- 8 oz minced lean beef

Vegetables

- 10 lb tomatoes
- 10 oz onions
- 14 oz carrots
- 4 lb turnips
- 1.5 lb radish
- 1 lb sweet potatoes
- 1 lb spinach
- 1 lb kale
- 4 bell peppers
- 24 oz cauliflower
- 9 oz broccoli (tenderstem)
- 6 leeks
- 1 lb lettuce
- 1 bunch of collard greens
- 14 ribs of celery
- 8 shallots
- 2 heads of garlic
- 2-inch piece of ginger
- 8 lemons
- 1 scallion
- 2 shallots

Fruits

- 4 avocado
- 2 pear
- 1 oz olives
- 8 oz fresh blueberries

Dairy

- cheese
- feta cheese
- parmesan
- 1 lb cream

Oil

- coconut oil
- canola oil
- vegetable oil

Butter

- 6 oz butter

Honey

- honey

Sugar

- small bag sugar

Nuts

- crushed peanuts
- walnuts

Seasoning and Flavors

- bay leaves
- cumin
- smoked paprika
- chili powder
- sage leaves
- turmeric
- mint
- parsley
- fresh dill
- thyme
- rosemary
- basil
- coriander
- flakes of red pepper
- wholegrain mustard
- 4 stemmed, seeded, minced serrano chiles
- apple cider vinegar

Others

- mild harissa
- dried marjoram
- Tabasco according to taste
- crusty bread
- breadcrumbs
- capers
- white wine
- rocket

- tamari
- rice vinegar (brown rice)
- reduced salt bouillon powder (vegetable)
- prepared ginger-sesame dressing

Kitchen Tools

- Dishtowel
- Pans and pots
- Can opener
- Mixing bowls
- Paper towels
- Whisks
- Strainer
- Spatulas
- A heavy pot
- Muffin tins
- Foil
- Baking Sheets
- Stick blender
- Brush
- Non-stick saucepan
- Parchment paper
- Measuring spoons and cups
- Cooling rack
- Stick blender
- Food processor
- Oven

Now that you know what ingredients and tools you will need let's get to the good part of the book - the recipes. You will find a variety of tasty recipes for breakfast in the next chapter. Best of all, they only take 30 minutes or less to make so you will have plenty of time to do other things too.

Chapter 8: Breakfast Recipes

Are you looking for a secret formula to be happier, healthier, and more productive in spite of being diabetic? You should start your day with a healthy breakfast.

To put it in simple words, food can influence a person's overall wellbeing. There are plenty of stories of individuals who could overcome their symptoms by just changing the foods that they ate.

The recipes that are given here contain eggs, salmon, avocado, cottage cheese, almonds, and chia seeds which are some excellent foods for diabetes. They make you feel full for longer and prevent overeating and weight gain. Above all, they do not raise glucose levels.

Turkey Rolls

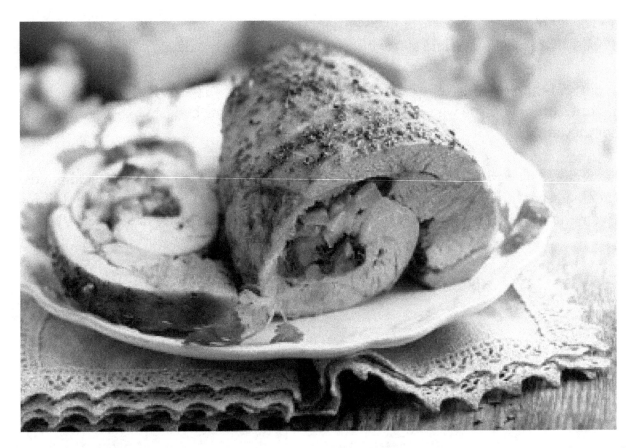

They are actually breadless sandwich wraps in which slices of turkey are wrapped around food items that have fewer carbs such as veggies and cheese.

They are a good option for people with diabetes because they offer more protein and fewer carbs. A roll gives around 5 g of protein. This is suitable for preventing glucose levels from shooting up.

Besides this, the protein present in the rolls can help to reduce your appetite. This, in turn, can prevent overeating and promote better management of weight. Both these factors are important for controlling diabetes mellitus type 2.

Time: 5 minutes

Serves: 1

Nutritional Facts: 155 Calories | 4.5 g Fats | 7.5 g Carbs | 22.9 g Protein

Ingredients

- 1 turkey slice
- 1 tbsp cream cheese
- 1/4 cucumber
- 1/2 bell pepper
- salt and seasoning according to taste

Procedure

1. Take a turkey slice and spread cream cheese on it.
2. Cut the cucumber and bell pepper into thin slices or pieces.
3. Place them on the layer of cheese.
4. Sprinkle some salt and seasoning.
5. Roll up the turkey slice and enjoy.

Low Carb Egg Bowl

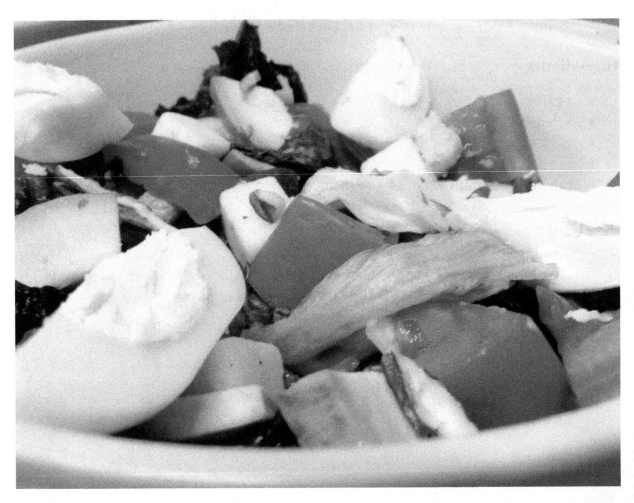

Eggs are very healthy for diabetic people. They contain 5.5 grams of protein which keeps you full and prevents the blood glucose from rising quickly.

A study was conducted in which 65 people with T2D participated. They ate 2 eggs every day for a period of 12 weeks. In the end, it was found that there was a significant reduction in fasting blood glucose levels for all of them. Their hemoglobin A1c was also lower (Elliott, 2018).

Time: 15 minutes

Serves: 2

Nutritional Facts: 178 Calories | 14.3 g Fats | 7.6 g Carbs | 6.9 g Protein

Ingredients

- 2 eggs
- 1/2 avocado
- 1/2 red onion
- 1/2 bell pepper
- Pepper and salt, to taste

Procedure

1. Put the eggs in a saucepan and pour some water in it. The water level should be 1" above the eggs. Place the saucepan on the stovetop and cover it. Boil the eggs on high heat for 7 minutes.
2. Take them out and put them in cold water. After they are cool enough to be handled, tap ~~Tap~~ on one end with the back part of a fork or spoon. Gently remove the outer shell. Cut into pieces.
3. Peel and cut avocado into small pieces.
4. Chop bell pepper and onion finely.
5. Combine avocado, eggs, bell pepper, and onion in one bowl.
6. Sprinkle pepper and salt.
7. Mix well and serve (Mullins, 2015).

Tasty Salmon Wrap

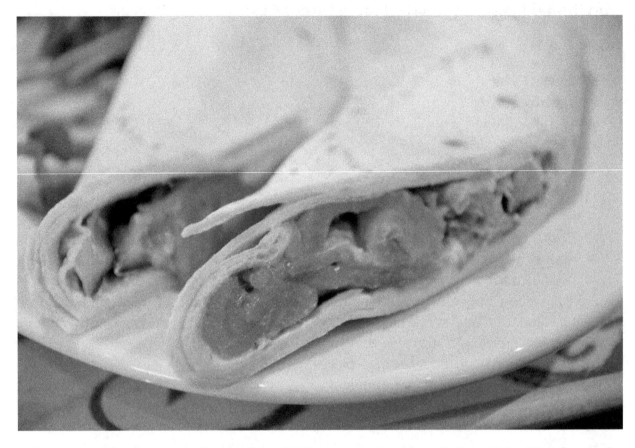

Salmon contains omega-3 fatty acids which protect the outer lining of the blood vessels, improve the functioning of the arteries, and reduce inflammation.

Many studies have shown that those people who consume fatty fish on a regular basis have less risk of suffering from heart failure.

Besides this, salmon also provides plenty of high-quality protein.

Time: 30 minutes

Serves: 4

Nutritional Facts: 362 Calories | 19.5 g Fats | 27 g Carbs | 23.1 g Protein

Ingredients

- 6 flour tortillas
- 14 oz salmon (smoked)
- 1 cup salmon flavored cream cheese
- 12 peppers (piquant)
- 1 avocado (sliced)
- 1 pear (sliced)
- 1/3 cucumber (chop into small sticks)
- Onion sprouts (sliced)

Procedure

1. Spread a layer of cream cheese on the tortillas. Arrange the peppers, avocado, pear, cucumber, and salmon in the center.
2. Sprinkle the onion sprouts and roll the tortillas. Use some cream cheese to seal the corners.
3. You can cut the rolls in half diagonally before serving.

Note:
You can find smoked salmon in the seafood section of the grocery shops. It is usually available in vacuum-sealed packets. You can buy Big Sam's Salmon Smoked - Pre-sliced, Trader Joe's Smoked Salmon or Norwegian Smoked Salmon for this recipe.

Carrot Hummus

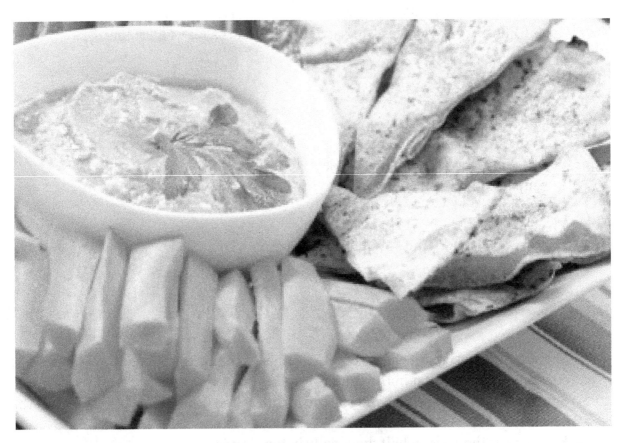

This recipe is very suitable for those who have diabetes because it contains ingredients like olive oil, almond butter, garlic, and lemon juice.

You already know that olive oil is beneficial for the heart since it has oleic acid that is monounsaturated fat which improves HDL and triglycerides. In addition, it may increase GLP-1, the hormone that makes you feel full.Nuts are very healthy for diabetic people. They contain fewer digestible carbohydrates and help to reduce the levels of insulin, blood sugar, and LDL cholesterol. You can gain this benefit as almond butter has been added in it.

Time required: 15 minutes

Serves: 4

Nutritional Facts: 168 Calories | 9 g Fats | 19.2 g Carbs | 4.5 g Protein

Ingredients

- 1 oz olive oil
- 1/2 oz almond butter
- 1 teaspoon honey
- 1 teaspoon cumin (ground)
- 1 teaspoon coriander (ground)
- 4 oz water
- 1 garlic clove
- 6 oz carrots (chopped into 1" pieces, roasted and cooled)
- 1 tablespoon lemon juice
- 2 oz chickpeas (canned, drained)
- 4 slices pita bread

Procedure

1. Put all the ingredients in the food processor to make the hummus.
2. Then serve with pita bread (Carrot Hummus, n.d.).

Avocado Toast

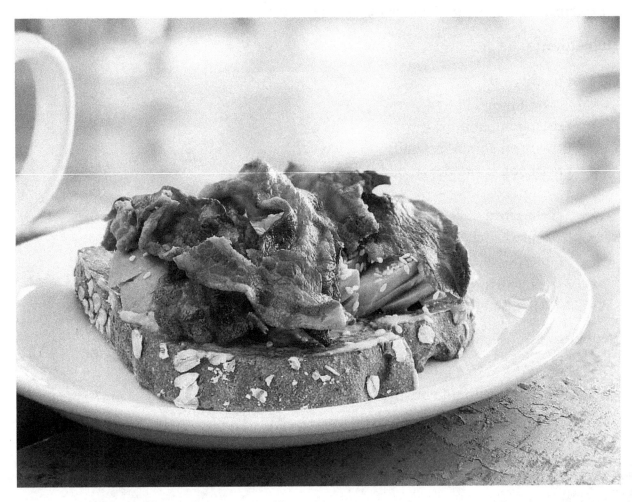

This is an excellent recipe for people with diabetes because avocado is its main ingredient. Avocados are remarkable plant sources of unsaturated fats which are the healthiest types of fats.

Besides this, lime juice has been used, which makes this dish more beneficial for people with diabetes. Research shows that oranges, lemons, grapefruits, and other citrus fruits have antidiabetic effects.

Time required: 10 minutes

Serves: 4

Nutritional Facts: 339 Calories | 27.9 g Fats | 15.2 g Carbs | 9.7 g Protein

Ingredients

- 2 avocados (peeled, pit removed)
- 4 bacon slices (cooked, cooled)
- 1 tablespoon lime juice (fresh)
- 1/3 teaspoon salt
- 1/3 teaspoon pepper (ground)
- 1/2 oz sriracha sauce
- 4 bread slices (whole wheat, toasted)

Procedure

1. Place the cooked and cooled bacon in the food processor and pulse three times. Then transfer the bacon to one small bowl.
2. Put the sriracha, avocado, lime juice, pepper, and salt in the jar. Then pulse around 7 times. After that, run it continuously for about 20 seconds.
3. Put around 2 tablespoons of chopped bacon and avocado spread on the toasted bread slices and serve (Avocado Toast, n.d.).

Note:

- Do not put hot ingredients in the blender.

Chia Pudding

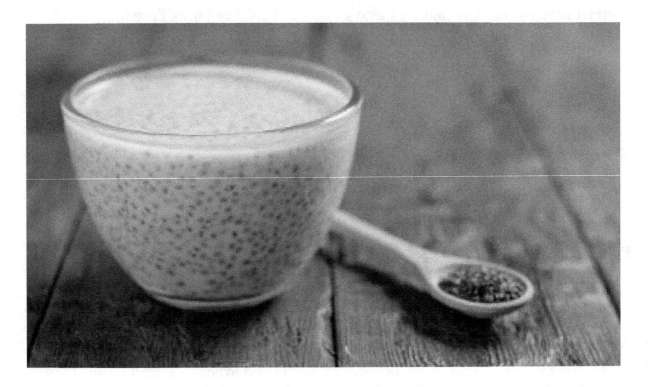

Chia seeds contain nutrients like omega 3 fats, protein, and fiber that help to stabilize blood glucose levels. The fiber in the seeds has the ability to absorb quite a lot of water. This can slow down digestion and the transfer of glucose to the blood, which can help to control diabetes.

Moreover, triglyceride levels can be lowered by eating these seeds, which is good for the heart. This is very useful for people with diabetes because they have a greater risk of getting heart disease.

Time: 5 minutes (soak for some time)

Serves: 1

Nutritional Facts: 155 Calories | 8 g Fats | 16 g Carbs | 4 g Protein

Ingredients

- 1 oz chia seeds
- 4 oz almond milk
- 1 tsp honey

Procedure

1. Put all the ingredients in a jar. Mix well. Allow them to settle for a few minutes. Mix them once again until all the clumps disappear.
2. Put a lid on the jar. Store it in the refrigerator for 2 hours or leave it overnight.
3. You can put some fresh fruits on top of the pudding when you eat it.

Note:

- You may use any variety of milk and sweetener according to your choice. All sorts of berries, such as strawberries and blueberries or any other fruits, can be used to make the topping.
- You can store the pudding in Tupperware or one mason jar for nearly a week in your refrigerator.
- Chia seeds are available in almost all big grocery stores. You can find them with the superfoods or in the cereal section.

Paleo Carrot and Pumpkin Muffins

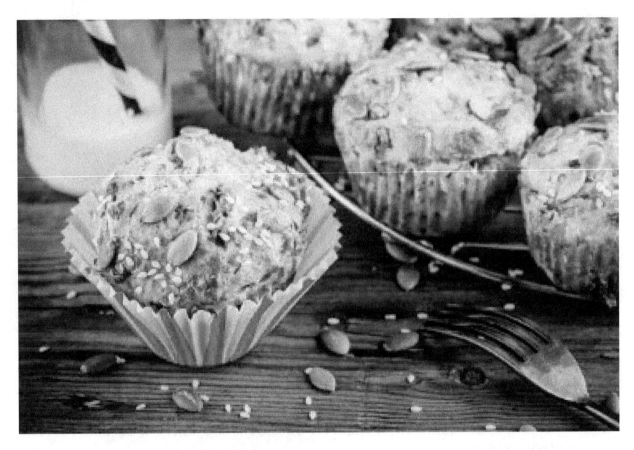

The muffins contain eggs which are great sources of protein. They reduce inflammation, increase good or HDL cholesterol, and improve the body's sensitivity to insulin. The veggies also provide plenty of fiber.

Besides this, cinnamon is used in this recipe which is a tasty spice as well as a powerful antioxidant. Several studies show that it can lower the levels of blood sugar and improve the body's insulin sensitivity.

Time: 30 minutes

Serves: 12 muffins

Nutritional Facts: 185 Calories | 11 g Fats | 19 g Carbs | 6 g Protein

Ingredients

- 3 eggs
- 4 carrots (peeled)
- 12 oz almond flour
- 2 tsp 5 spice powder
- 1 tsp baking soda
- 2 tbsp almond butter
- 1/2 tsp tartaric acid
- 1/2 tsp cinnamon (ground)
- 1/2 tsp sea salt
- 4 oz honey
- 6 oz pumpkin puree (canned)
- 1 tbsp almonds (sliced)
- 1 tbsp pumpkin seeds (toasted)
- 1 tsp coconut oil (some extra oil for greasing muffin tin in case you are not using the paper liners)

Tools required

- oven
- muffin tin
- paper liners
- food processor
- mixing bowls
- dish towel

Procedure

1. Heat the oven to a temperature of 350 degrees Fahrenheit. Take out the eggs from the fridge, so they are at room temperature by the time you blend the ingredients. Put the paper liners in the cups of a ~~and line one~~ muffin tin.

2. Grate the carrots with a food processor or by hand. Put them in a dish towel ~~Gather its sides~~ and squeeze out the extra liquid. ~~carrot juice.~~ Set aside the shredded carrot. There should be one and a half cups of finely shredded carrots for this recipe.

3. Whisk the 5-spice powder, almond flour, baking soda, ground cinnamon, sea salt and tartaric acid in one large bowl.

4. Beat the eggs in another bowl.

5. Mix the pumpkin, almond butter, coconut oil and honey in a separate bowl. These ingredients should be at normal room temperature; otherwise the coconut oil may harden and form lumps. Make sure that the batter is smooth.

6. Mix the wet items with the dry ingredients in the large bowl and stir well.

7. Add the shredded carrots.

8. Fill the batter equally in each cup of the muffin tin. Each cup should be 3/4th full.

9. Sprinkle the pumpkin seeds and sliced almonds on top. Then place the muffin tin in the oven.

10. Bake the muffins at 375 degrees F for thirty minutes. Rotate the tin containing the muffins 180 degrees when they are half cooked.

11. You can test if the muffins are ready by inserting a toothpick in them. If the toothpick is clean when you take it out, the muffins are done. You can also know that they are done if they are springy when touching them.

12. Take out the muffin tin and let it cool for five minutes.

13. Remove the muffins from the tray, place them on a rack and cool them completely.

Chapter 9: Soups and Stews

Soups and stews are great mood boosters. They offer physical as well as emotional warmth. The most important thing is that they are less prone to spiking your glucose levels.

However, many times people find it difficult to come up with novel ideas for making healthy soups which are low in carbs. It is easy to find recipes for losing weight, getting rid of belly fat, or eating a gluten-free diet. But there are not many sources that specifically cater to the diabetic diet.

Here you will find a variety of delicious recipes which will not only satiate your cravings but also offer a treat to your palate.

Arctic Char Soup

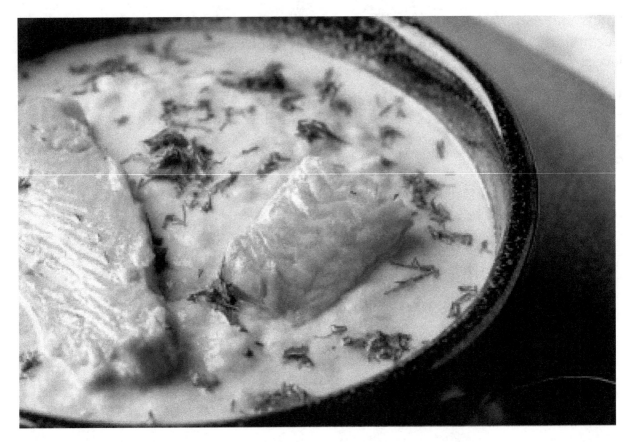

Fatty fish is considered to be a very healthy food item and is highly recommended for people with diabetes. Salmon is a fatty fish which is the key ingredient of this soup. It is an excellent source of omega-3 fats EPA and DHA, which are extremely beneficial for the heart.

Consuming enough healthy fats is important for people with diabetes as they have a greater risk of experiencing a stroke and heart disease.

Time: 30 minutes

Serves: 4

Nutritional Facts: 535 Calories | 30.9 g Fats | 15.1 g Carbs | 8.4 g Protein

Ingredients

- 24 oz Arctic Char (wild salmon, thick fillets are preferable as it is easier to cut them into cubes)
- 28 oz can of crushed tomatoes (without added salt)
- 2 oz butter
- 1 bay leaf
- 4 oz each of onion, carrots, celery (chopped)
- 4 oz heavy cream (optional)
- 1/4 teaspoon thyme
- 8 oz vegetable broth
- Pepper and salt to taste

Tools required

- a heavy pot

Procedure

1. Remove all the bones and the skin of the fish. You can use a sharp knife's tip to do this or get it done in the shop itself.
2. Cut the fillets into three-fourth inch cubes. Put some pepper and salt on them.
3. Melt the butter in one heavy pot on medium heat. Add the onion, carrots, and celery — Cook for five minutes. Then put in the broth, thyme, bay leaf and tomatoes.
4. Cover it and allow it to simmer for fifteen minutes. Add the fillets and the cream. Stir to mix the cream properly. Cover it or simmer without covering the vessel for ten to fifteen more minutes. Stir occasionally.
5. Take out the bay leaf, check and adjust the seasoning if needed. You can add some fresh herbs like thyme for more flavor.

Turkey, Cauliflower and Kale Soup

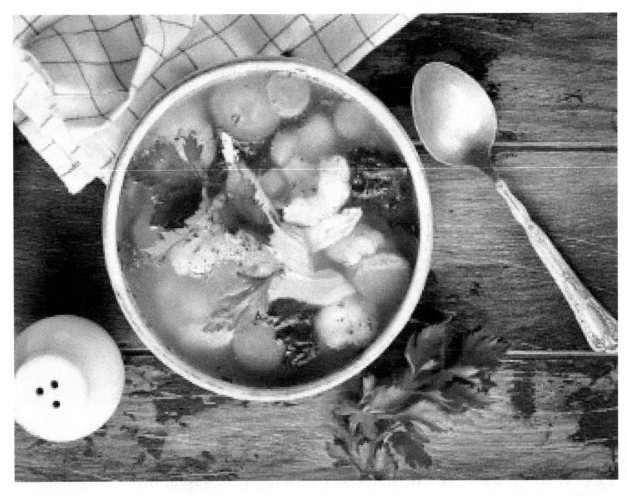

This recipe is very special because all its chief components, namely turkey, cauliflower, and kale, are diabetes friendly.

White skinless turkey is a good choice for people with diabetes because it contains less fat and more protein.

Cauliflower is a low carbohydrate vegetable which is a boon for diabetic meal plans. It is a rich source of vitamin C and also provides folate, potassium, and fiber.

Kale contains numerous essential minerals and vitamins. It has vitamin C, which helps in reducing fasting blood glucose levels and inflammatory markers.

Best of all, you can make this tasty, nutritious soup in less than 30 minutes.

Time: 30 minutes

Serves: 4

Nutritional Facts: 356 Calories | 13.3 g Fats | 21.7 g Carbs | 39 g Protein

Ingredients

- 3 carrots (cut into slices)
- 1 pound turkey (ground)
- 4 shallots (cut into pieces)
- 1 capsicum (chopped into pieces)
- 4 cups of chicken stock
- 15 ounce can of tomatoes (diced)
- 4 cups of kale (without ribs, leaves chopped coarsely)
- 12 oz cauliflower (minced)
- 2 tablespoons of coconut oil
- Sea salt
- Black pepper (freshly ground)

Procedure

1. Place a saucepan on medium to high heat and melt the coconut oil.
2. Add the carrots, capsicum, shallots, and cauliflower.
3. Cook for eight to ten minutes until the veggies become slightly soft. Stir frequently.
4. Add in the turkey and cook for six to eight minutes until it is cooked properly.
5. Then add in the chicken stock, and diced tomatoes. Season with pepper and salt according to taste.
6. Allow the contents to start boiling. Mix the kale, reduce the heat, cover the pan and allow it to simmer for fifteen minutes. After it's done, ladle the soup in a bowl and enjoy.

Healthy Escarole and Chicken Soup

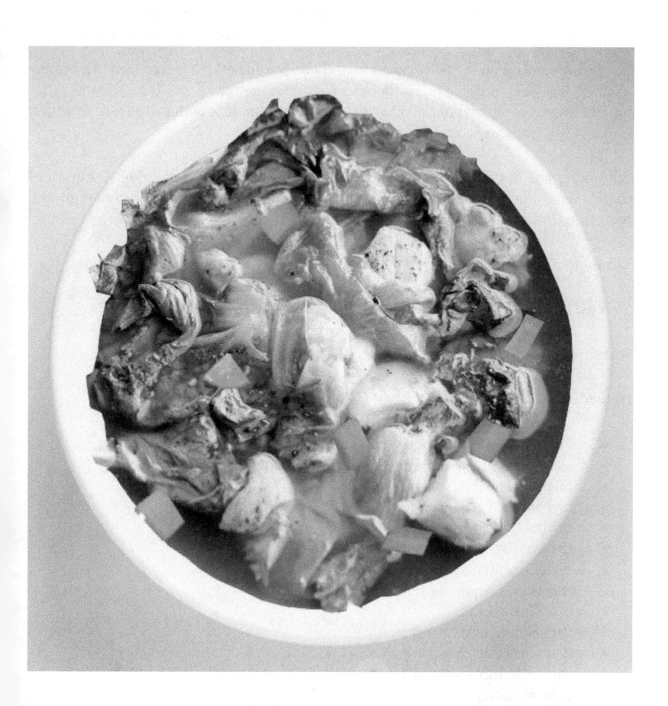

This soup recipe is packed full of healthy ingredients like escarole, chicken, and olive oil. Escarole offers many nutritional benefits, such as folate, fiber, and minerals. This fantastic green has very few carbs and calories. In order to enjoy all the benefits of this veggie, buy the ones that have green and crisp leaves, and heads that are firmly packed.

Chicken is rich in protein and is a good food choice for diabetics if it is cooked in a healthy manner. It is best to use skinless, boneless, chicken breasts as much as possible. They contain less fat compared to the other parts of a chicken. It is better to substitute butter with olive oil when you cook chicken on a stovetop.

Olive oil is one of the healthiest oils for your heart. It contains antioxidants known as polyphenols. They decrease the levels of blood pressure, reduce inflammation, and protect the lining of the blood vessels.

Time: 30 minutes

Serves: 4

Nutritional Facts: 542 Calories | 22.6 g Fats | 23.5 g Carbs | 60.9 g Protein

Ingredients

- 28 oz chicken breasts (boneless, skinless)
- 2 leeks (light green and white parts cut into half circles quarter-inch thick)
- 2 tbsp olive oil (extra virgin)
- 2 ribs of celery (chopped into half-inch pieces)
- 3 carrots (chopped into half-inch pieces)
- 1 can (14.5 oz) of diced tomatoes
- 2 cloves of garlic (chopped)
- 1/4 tsp black pepper (ground)
- 3/4 tsp kosher salt
- 2 tbsp lemon juice (fresh)
- 2 tbsp fresh dill (chopped)
- 4 cups of lettuce (chopped)
- 8 cups of water

Procedure

1. Heat oil on medium to high heat and sauté the leeks for five minutes until they become tender.
2. Add in the celery, carrots, and garlic. Cook for five minutes stirring frequently.
3. Add in the water, tomatoes, pepper, and salt.
4. Then add the chicken breasts and allow the contents to start boiling. Reduce the heat and simmer for fifteen minutes.
5. Take out the chicken and place it on one cutting surface or plate. When it becomes cool, take a fork and shred it. Put the shredded chicken back in the soup pot.
6. Add the escarole and simmer for two to three minutes. Mix the lemon juice. Serve the soup in bowls and sprinkle some dill.

Nachos Soup

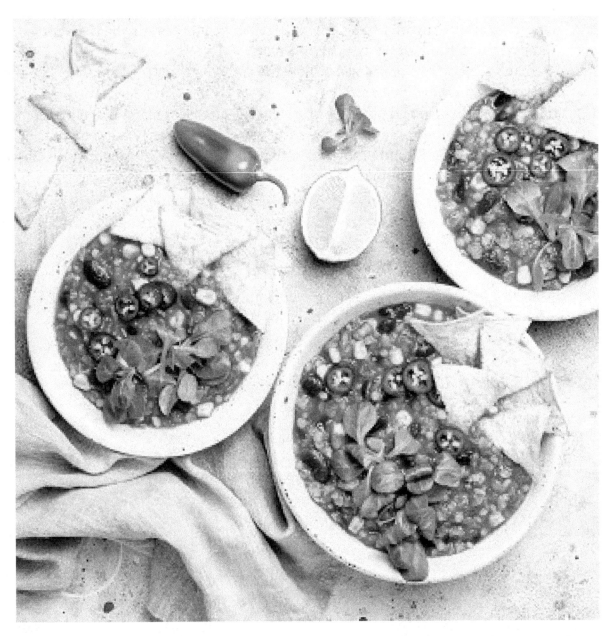

This nacho soup takes only 30 minutes to make and is packed full of healthy ingredients, such as onions, cumin, paprika, and kidney beans. Beans provide an abundant amount of protein and help you to feel full longer. In this way, eating beans can be helpful in shedding the extra pounds. It can also help to regulate the levels of cholesterol and blood pressure.

When using canned beans, choose beans which do not contain added salt or rinse them before using.

Time: 30 minutes

Serves: 4

Nutritional Facts: 339 Calories | 20.7 g Fats | 26.9 g Carbs | 16.4 g Protein

Ingredients

- 1 tbsp olive oil
- 4 oz minced lean beef
- 1 clove of garlic (chopped finely)
- 1 onion (chopped)
- 1 tbsp cumin (ground)
- 1 tbsp coriander (ground)
- 2 tsp smoked paprika
- 1 tbsp chili powder
- 4 oz tomatoes (chopped)
- 4 oz tomato puree
- 1.5 cups of chicken stock
- 1 oz corn (whole kernel)
- 1 oz kidney beans
- 1 oz cream
- 1 tsp sugar
- Pepper
- Salt
- 1 oz grated cheddar cheese
- A handful of coriander or basil leaves
- 1 avocado (diced)

Procedure

1. Heat the oil in one soup pot on medium heat. Sauté the onions in it for two minutes.
2. Add the garlic and minced beef and fry for eight minutes.
3. Put the cumin, paprika, chili powder, coriander, and sugar in it — Fry for two minutes.
4. Then put in the chopped tomatoes, chicken stock, corn, tomato puree, and beans and simmer for ten minutes. Add in the cream. Adjust the seasoning if needed.
5. Ladle the soup into serving bowls. Put some avocado and cheese on top. Garnish with coriander or basil leaves and serve.

Sweet Potato and Harissa Soup

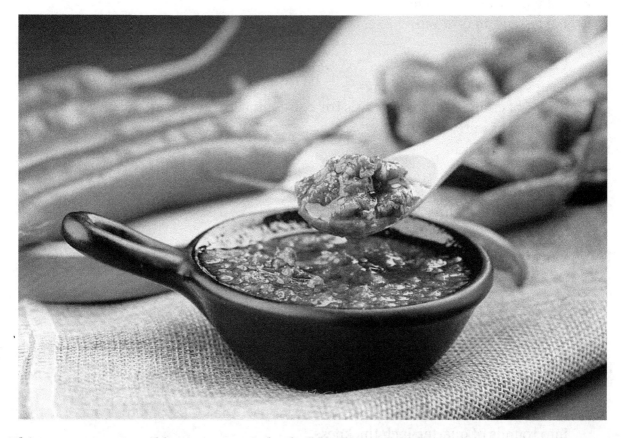

This sweet potato and harissa soup is both delicious and feeling. Sweet potatoes occupy a lower position on the GI scale compared to white potatoes. So, they are a good choice for diabetic people.

Time: 30 minutes

Serves: 4

Nutritional Facts: 215 Calories | 11.5 g Fats | 22.5 g Carbs | 7.8 g Protein

Ingredients

- 8 oz sweet potatoes
- 1/2 onion (yellow)
- 1 tbsp olive oil
- 1/2 tsp turmeric (ground)
- 1/2 tsp cumin (ground)
- 1 clove of garlic
- 1 oz tomato paste
- 2 cups of vegetable broth
- 2 cups of chopped spinach leaves (or baby spinach)
- 3/4 cups of water
- 1/4 tsp kosher salt
- 1 oz peanut butter
- Mild harissa
- 1 oz crushed peanuts

Tools required

- heavy pan
- immersion blender

Procedure

1. Dice the onion, mince the cloves of garlic, peel the sweet potatoes and cut them into rounds of quarter-inch thickness.
2. Heat a tablespoon of olive oil on medium to high heat in a big heavy-bottomed pan. Add the onion. Sauté for five to seven minutes.
3. Add the tomato paste, peanut butter, turmeric, garlic, and cumin. Cook for one-minute stirring constantly.
4. Put the sweet potatoes, water, and vegetable broth in the pan. Simmer for 20 to 25 minutes on medium to low heat.
5. After the sweet potatoes become soft, blend all the contents with the help of an immersion blender. Add half a teaspoon of kosher salt. Let the soup simmer once again. Put spinach leaves in the pan and cook for one minute.
6. Garnish with harissa and crushed peanuts. Serve in bowls with toasted bread slices.

Pumpkin and Lentil Soup

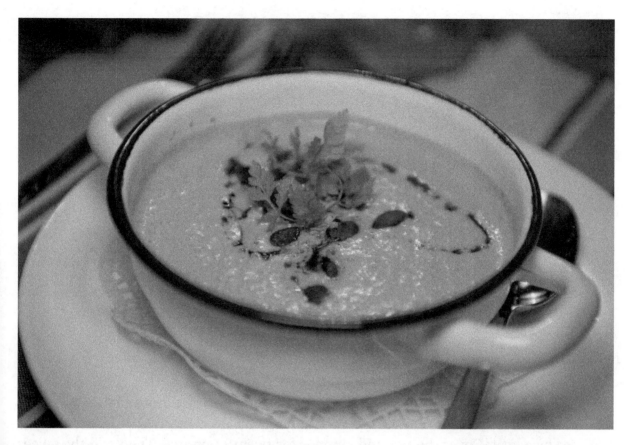

You can gain a lot of health benefits from this recipe. Pumpkin is packed with nutrients that help in controlling blood sugar. It can also slow down the progression of diabetes in certain cases. The entire pumpkin, even its leaves and seeds have less sugar and more nutrients. Pumpkin extract can have an insulin-like effect.

Red lentil is the other chief ingredient for this dish. Lentils have soluble fiber which helps to stabilize blood glucose levels.

Time: 30 minutes

Serves: 4

Nutritional Facts: 128 Calories | 1 g Fats | 20.8 g Carbs | 9.2 g Protein

Ingredients

- 1/2 big onion (chopped)
- 1 clove of garlic (diced)
- 1 carrot (cut into pieces)
- 1 rib of celery (chopped)
- 1/2 cup of red lentils
- 4 oz pumpkin (without sugar)
- 2 cups of vegetable broth
- 1/8 tsp dried thyme
- 1/8 tsp dried marjoram
- Tabasco according to taste

Procedure

1. Mix the garlic, onion, carrots, celery, lentils, and water or broth in one pot. Heat the pot and allow the contents to start boiling.
2. Reduce heat. Cover the pot and simmer for twenty minutes. Then add the spices and pumpkin. Simmer until the contents are thoroughly blended. Add tabasco according to taste and serve.

Sprouted Lentils with Vegan Stew

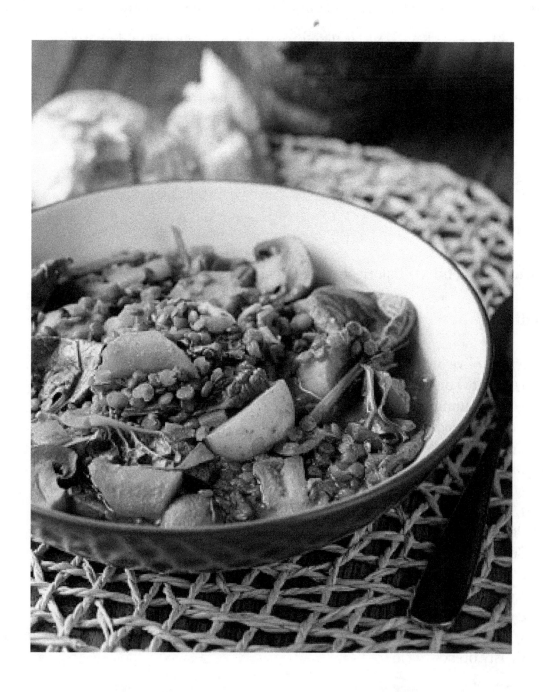

This is a fantastic recipe which is tasty and nutritious. It includes lentils which contain 25% protein and have a low glycemic index. So, they are ideal for diabetic meals and can be eaten regularly. In fact, pulse consumption can reduce the chances of getting diabetes.

Even though carrots have a sweet flavor, they can be included in diabetic meals because they can help to manage blood sugar levels.

Tomatoes also have a low glycemic index and have fewer calories and are non-starchy. Besides this, onions are included in the recipe, which can also help to control blood glucose.

Time: 30 minutes

Serves: 4

Nutritional Facts: 211 Calories | 7.6 g Fats | 27.1 g Carbs | 10.1 g Protein

Ingredients

- 2 tbsp olive oil (extra virgin)
- 1/2 yellow onion
- 1/2 tsp cumin (ground)
- 1 carrot (medium size)
- 1 clove of garlic
- 1 rib of celery
- 1/4 tsp coriander (ground)
- 1/8 tsp flakes of red pepper
- Pepper (ground)
- Sea salt
- 2 cups of vegetable stock
- 5 oz package of green lentils (sprouted)
- 8 oz of diced tomatoes
- 1/2 bunch of Tuscan kale (chopped into bite-size pieces without the tough stems)
- Crusty bread

Procedure

1. Cut the onion, carrots, and celery. Mince the garlic.
2. Heat olive oil in one heavy-bottomed pan on medium to high heat. Add the onion, celery, and carrots and sauté them for three minutes. Stir occasionally. Add the garlic and cook for one more minute. Then add the coriander, cumin, and flakes of red pepper and sauté for two minutes — season with pepper and salt.
3. Add the vegetable stock, lentils, and tomatoes and allow the contents to start boiling. Then lower the heat and simmer for twenty to twenty-five minutes until the mixture thickens. Put the kale and let it simmer for one or two minutes. Check the taste and add pepper and salt.
4. Serve the stew and crusty bread together.

Chapter 10: Tasty and Healthy Recipes

This section has been specially designed to meet the requirements of the diabetic diet. It is packed with recipes to help improve your overall health and keep your blood sugar levels in check. Just pick up a few recipes each day, give a boost to your body, and march ahead towards your goal of managing or even reversing diabetes.

Roasted Beet, Pear and Walnut Salad

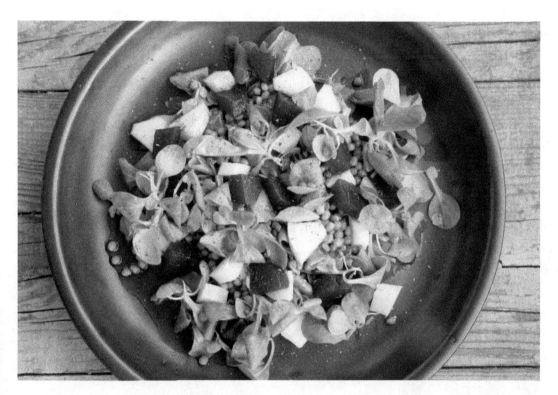

This amazing dish is prepared with some of the most nutritious ingredients. Beetroot can help to reduce the risk of various diabetes complications, such as eye and nerve damage. They also contain phytochemicals which have a regulating impact on insulin and glucose.

Pears contain a lot of fiber and have a significant amount of vitamin K. They are a good choice for those who have diabetes because they have a low glycemic index.

Walnuts contain healthy fatty acids, such as alpha-lipoic, which are good for the heart. If a person has diabetes, there is a greater risk of getting a stroke or heart disease. So, it is good to include the sources of such fatty acids in the diet.

Time: 30 minutes

Serves: 4

Nutritional Facts: 438 Calories | 28.2 g Fats | 34.9 g Carbs | 16.2 g Protein

Ingredients

- 3 beets (medium size)
- 1 pear (cut into half-inch pieces)
- 4 oz walnuts (toasted)
- Some salad greens
- 4 oz feta cheese
- 4 oz cooked quinoa
- Micro sprouts (optional)
- 1 tablespoon each of olive oil, walnut oil, balsamic vinegar, and honey
- Black pepper
- Sea salt

Tools required

- oven
- foil

Procedure

1. Heat the oven to a temperature of 350 degrees. Put the beets on a plate. Drizzle some olive oil on the beets and sprinkle pepper and salt on them. Wrap them in foil, place them on a baking tray and roast them for about 15 to 20 minutes. The time will depend on the size of the beets.
2. Let them cool. When they are sufficiently cool, put them under running water and slide their skins off by hand. Chop them into half-inch cubes. Keep them aside and let them cool completely.
3. Arrange the beets, pear, walnuts, salad greens, feta cheese, cooked quinoa, and micro sprouts on a plate. Drizzle some olive oil, walnut oil, balsamic vinegar, and honey on them. Sprinkle some pepper and salt on top. Serve it along with fried rice or pasta.

Chicken Salad with Ginger and Sesame Dressing

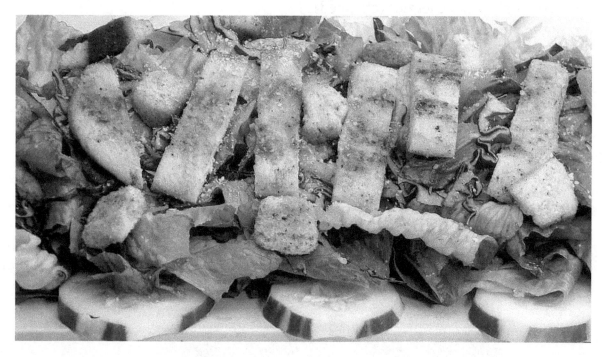

This healthy, delicious salad takes only 30 minutes to make. Besides chicken breasts, it contains spinach and romaine lettuce. These leafy green vegetables are nutritious and have fewer digestible carbs which can raise blood sugar levels. They also contain the antioxidants zeaxanthin and lutein that protect the eyes from cataracts and macular degeneration which are some common complications associated with diabetes.

Time: 30 minutes

Serves: 4

Nutritional Facts: 71 Calories | 1.1 g Fats | 9.6 g Carbs | 6.6 g Protein

Ingredients

- 3 oz chicken breast (shredded, cooked)
- 4 cups of romaine lettuce (chopped)
- 4 oz spinach (fresh)
- 2 oz carrot (shredded)
- 10 oz radish (sliced)
- 1 scallion (cut into slices)
- 3 tbsp prepared ginger-sesame dressing

Procedure

1. Combine the chicken, lettuce, spinach, radishes, scallion, and carrots into one bowl.
2. Add the prepared ginger-sesame dressing.
3. Toss the contents, so it mixes well with the dressing. You can serve it with rice or noodles.

Tuna Salad Mediterranean Style

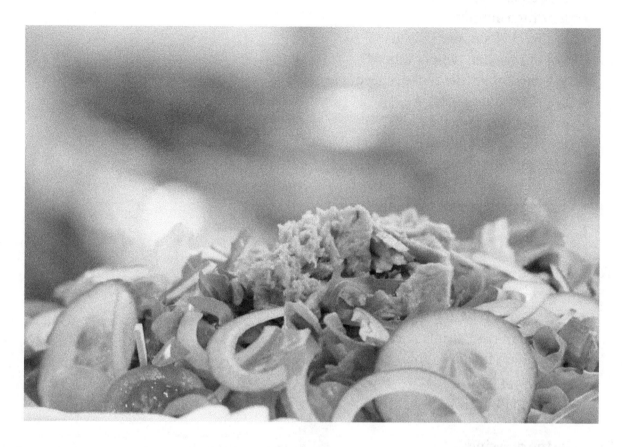

This salad contains tuna which is extremely healthy for people with diabetes since it's low in carbs. For example, 3 oz of tuna has no carbs but provides 22 g of protein. Besides this, it's high in omega 3 fats which help in managing diabetes. As discussed, omega 3 fats help to improve the regulation of blood sugar and reduce inflammation.

Time: 30 minutes

Serves: 4

Nutritional Facts: 183 Calories | 6.1 g Fats | 22.5 g Carbs | 10.9 g Protein

Ingredients

- 4 oz chickpeas
- 2 oz tuna chunks
- 1/4 red bell pepper (sliced)
- 1/4 orange bell pepper (sliced)
- 1/2 cucumber (deseeded, sliced)
- 1/4 tbsp capers
- 1 oz feta (crumbled)
- 2 oz cherry tomatoes (cut into halves)
- 1/2 scallion (sliced thinly)
- 1/4 oz tomatoes (semi-sundried)
- 1/2 tsp parsley and fresh dill (chopped roughly)
- 1 oz olives (pitted)

To make the onion pickle:

- 1/2 teaspoon castor sugar
- 1/4 onion (red, thinly sliced)
- 1 oz cider vinegar (apple)
- 1/4 teaspoon salt
- Black pepper (ground)

To make the dressing:

- 1/2 tablespoon olive oil (extra virgin)
- 1/2 tablespoon lemon juice
- 1/2 teaspoon wholegrain mustard
- 1/4 teaspoon honey
- Pepper and salt according to taste

Procedure

1. First, make the pickle. Mix the vinegar, sugar, pepper, and salt in one bowl (non-metallic). When the sugar is dissolved, add the onions and keep aside for thirty minutes.
2. Put all the ingredients except the tuna in one big bowl to make the salad.
3. To make the dressing, whisk the ingredients mentioned above until the lemon juice and oil emulsify.
4. Pour this dressing on the salad. Toss to mix it properly. Then add the tuna chunks. Turn over gently so that the tuna does not break much.
5. Transfer the contents to one serving platter.
6. Take out the onions from the vinegar and spread on the salad. You can serve it with pasta or rice.

Chicken Meatballs

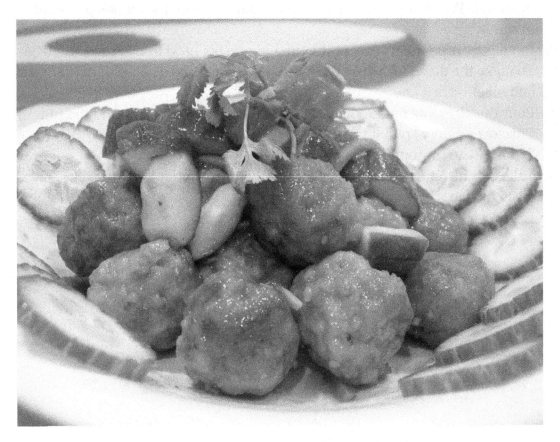

Chicken is a good source of protein, so are an excellent choice for a healthy meal. Canola oil has been included in this dish which contains healthy fatty acids like olives and avocados. This helps to reduce the bad cholesterol and blood glucose levels of diabetic people.

Besides this, this recipe uses sage leaves which are used as a remedy for diabetes.

Time: 30 minutes

Serves: 4

Nutritional Facts: 549 Calories | 30.6 g Fats | 24.2 g Carbs | 39.8 g Protein

Ingredients

- 12 oz minced chicken
- 1/2 onion (chopped finely)
- 3 tbsp sage leaves (chopped)
- 1 egg
- 2.5 oz breadcrumbs
- 1 lemon (grated zest)
- 3 ribs of celery
- 2 tbsp canola oil
- Sea salt
- White pepper
- 4 oz white wine
- 4 oz chicken stock
- 4 oz parmesan (grated)
- 8 oz cream
- Arugula

Procedure

1. Mix the minced chicken, onion, egg, sage, celery, salt, lemon zest, breadcrumbs, pepper, and salt in one bowl. Divide the mixture into 12 portions. Pick up each portion and roll it in your palm. In this way, make 12 balls with the mixture and put them in one baking tray that has been lined. Keep it in the refrigerator for ten minutes.
2. Heat some oil in one pan on the stovetop and fry the meatballs until they become golden brown. This may take about 10 to 15 minutes. Remove the meatballs and place them on one paper towel to get rid of the excess oil.
3. In the meantime, put the chicken stock, cream, and wine in a pan. Simmer the sauce until it becomes thick and is reduced in quantity. Put the meatballs in the pan and cook for a few minutes.
4. Garnish with grated parmesan and arugula. You can serve it with plain rice or slices of bread.

Teriyaki-Braised Greens and Turnips with Bacon

This is a tasty dish which has a number of health benefits. It contains leafy greens which provide vitamin C. Intake of vitamin C can reduce fasting blood glucose levels and inflammatory markers for people who have diabetes.

Turnips have plenty of fiber and help you to feel full longer. Eating more fiber can also help to keep blood glucose levels stable.

Ginger and garlic are included in this recipe. Ginger has a low glycemic index. Eating about 4 g of ginger daily can help in lowering blood glucose levels and regulating insulin production.

Garlic can help in managing blood sugar. Consumption of aged, raw, or cooked garlic can regulate blood sugar and reduce the impact of a few diabetes complications.

Keep in mind that this recipe contains bacon. Therefore, you should eat only a limited amount of bacon if you have diabetes because it has a lot of saturated fats.

Time: 30 minutes

Serves: 4

Nutritional Facts: 187 Calories | 4.3 g Fats | 29.4 g Carbs | 8.1 g Protein

Ingredients

To make the teriyaki sauce:

- 3 tablespoons tamari
- 1 tablespoon ginger (minced)
- 2 cloves of garlic (minced)
- 3 tablespoons rice vinegar (brown rice)
- 2 tablespoons honey

- 1/2 teaspoon pepper flakes

To make the main dish:

- 1 shallot (medium size, sliced thinly)
- 2 slices of bacon (nitrate free, cut into half-inch pieces)
- 1 bunch of collard greens (4 cups after cutting)
- 1 bunch of green onions
- 2 pounds of turnips (cut them into wedges)

Procedure

1. Mix the ingredients for the sauce in one small bowl.
2. Put the bacon in a pan with some fat. Place the pan on a stovetop and cook on low heat for 5 to 10 minutes until it becomes slightly brown.
3. Add in the shallots. Let them caramelize and allow the bacon to become crisp.
4. Increase the heat moderately and add the turnips. Let them turn brown on both sides.
5. Add the greens and the sauce. Cook on medium to high heat for ten minutes until the turnips become tender. Stir occasionally. Add the green onions.
6. The dish is ready to be served.

Broccoli and Barley Risotto with Basil and Lemon

This recipe contains broccoli which is a low-carb, low-calorie food. It is full of healthy compounds that protect against several diseases. Consuming broccoli can help in lowering insulin levels.

The other key ingredient is barley which has a low glycemic index. It does not cause as much change in the blood glucose levels as brown rice. It contains dietary fibers which can help to reduce an individual's appetite and also reduce the risk of getting cardiovascular disease.

Time: 30 minutes

Serves: 4

Nutritional Facts: 195 Calories | 7.6 g Fats | 28.9 g Carbs | 4.5 g Protein

Ingredients

- 4 oz pearl barley (whole grain)
- 2 teaspoons reduced-salt bouillon powder (vegetable)
- 1 leek (chopped)
- 1/2 teaspoon lemon juice (fresh)
- 2 tablespoons vegetable oil
- 2 cloves of garlic
- 2 tablespoons basil
- 4.5 oz broccoli (tenderstem)

Tools required

- stick blender
- non-stick saucepan
- mixing bowls

Procedure

1. Soak the barley in four cups of water, cover it, and leave it overnight.
2. Drain the grains and keep the liquid. Use it for making vegetable bouillon.
3. Then heat 1 tablespoon of oil in one non-stick saucepan. Put the leek in the pan and cook for 5 to 10 minutes until it softens. Take out half of the leek in one bowl. Add the bouillon and barley and cover the saucepan. Simmer for twenty minutes.
4. In the meantime, add the lemon juice, basil, garlic, three tablespoons of water, and the remaining oil to the bowl in which you have kept half of the leeks. Use a stick blender and blend these items to make a paste.
5. After cooking the barley for twenty minutes, add the broccoli. Cook for five to ten more minutes until they become tender. Add the leek puree and heat for 2 minutes. Then serve in bowls.

Blueberry and Avocado Salsa

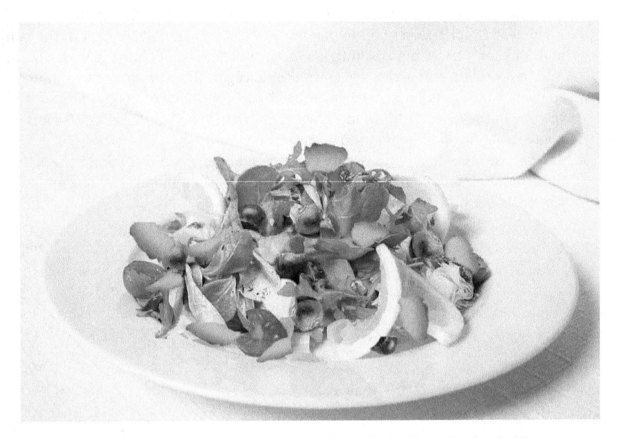

This tasty salsa takes 15 minutes to make and combines healthy foods like tomatoes, onions, chilies, blueberries, and avocado. Avocados have plenty of fiber and monounsaturated fats which makes them diabetes-friendly. These nutrients prevent blood glucose from rising quickly after meals. A study published in Diabetes Care, in 2016 showed that people who eat foods containing monounsaturated fats regularly show a significant improvement in their blood sugar levels.

Time: 15 minutes

Serves: 4

Nutritional Facts: 137 Calories | 10 g Fats | 12.5 g Carbs | 1.7 g Protein

Ingredients

- 2 diced red tomatoes
- 1/2 minced white onion
- 2 stemmed, seeded, minced serrano chiles
- 1 tablespoon minced fresh cilantro, basil, or mint
- 1 peeled, seeded, diced, ripe avocado
- 1/4 teaspoon sea salt
- 4 oz fresh blueberries

Procedure

1. Combine tomatoes, onion, serrano chiles, cilantro, avocado, blueberries, and sea salt in a large bowl.
2. Allow them to rest for a minimum of ten minutes so that the flavors can blend before serving.

You can refer to the next chapter to prepare various types of snacks, desserts, and smoothies while following the 14-day meal plan.

Chapter 11: Snacks, Desserts, and Drinks

It can be difficult to choose healthy snacks, desserts, and drinks when you have diabetes. The recipes given here will make this task easier. These food items contain nutrients that help to keep your sugar levels stable while also improving your overall health.

Yogurt and Berries

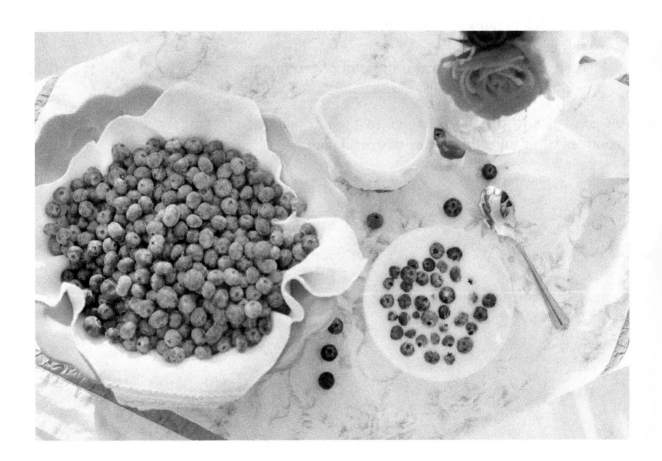

This is an awesome snack that only takes 5 minutes to make and is diabetes friendly.

Berries contain antioxidants that can decrease inflammation and save the pancreatic cells from damage. They are also rich in fiber, which slows down digestion and stabilizes sugar levels. For instance, 1 cup of blueberries gives about 4 g of fiber.

Yogurt also has probiotics that can improve the body's capacity to metabolize food items with sugar.

You can buy the plain, full fat, organic, or the grass-fed varieties of Greek yogurt. Some of the good quality brands that you can buy from are Wallaby Organic, Kalona Super Natural Organic, Maple Hill Creamery, and Redwood Hill Farms.

Time: 5 minutes

Serves: 1

Nutritional Facts: 216 Calories | 3.3 g Fats | 27.8 g Carbs | 14.5 g Protein

Ingredients

- ½ cup blueberries
- 1 cup yogurt (preferably Greek yogurt)

Procedure

1. Put the blueberries in a large bowl and wash them with tap water.
2. Take one medium-sized bowl.
3. Pour half a cup of yogurt in it.
4. Put a quarter cup of berries on the yogurt.
5. Pour the remaining yogurt.
6. Spread the rest of the berries on the layer of yogurt.

Peanut Butter and Apple

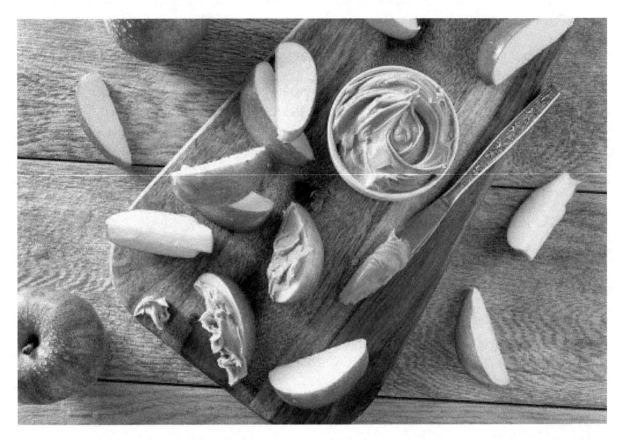

This tasty treat combines peanut butter and apples together, both of which are diabetes-friendly. Peanut butter contains plenty of manganese, magnesium, and vitamin E, while apples provide nutrients like potassium, vitamin B, and vitamin C. Moreover, both of them have a lot of fiber. You get 7 g of fiber when you combine 1 oz peanut butter with 1 medium-sized apple. This is useful for keeping blood glucose levels under control.

Time: 5 minutes

Serves: 1

Nutritional Facts: 105 Calories | 4.2 g Fats | 17 g Carbs | 2.3 g Protein

Ingredients

- 1/2 tbsp peanut butter
- 1/2 apple

Procedure

1. Wash the apple and cut it into small pieces.
2. Put the pieces into a bowl and put a little peanut butter on top of them. Serve and enjoy.

Roasted Chickpeas

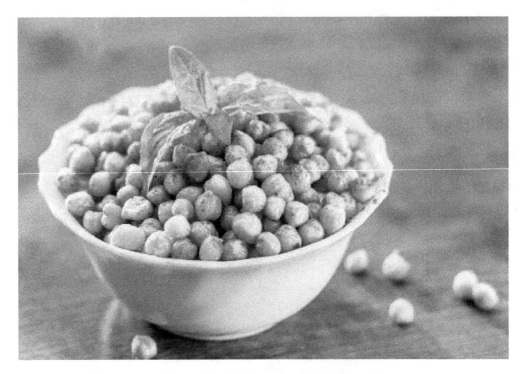

Chickpeas are also called garbanzo beans and are very healthy legumes. They provide a lot of fiber and protein, so they are excellent for people with diabetes.

Research shows that eating chickpeas regularly can help to prevent the advancement of diabetes because they have the capacity to help in the management of blood glucose levels.

A study was conducted with 19 adult participants who ate chickpea-based meals every day for 6 weeks. It was found that their insulin and blood sugar levels were much lower after eating than the individuals who consumed wheat-based meals (Elliott, 2018).

Time: 30 minutes

Serves: 4

Nutritional Facts: 89.5 Calories | 3.2 g Fats | 12.2 g Carbs | 3.7 g Protein

Ingredients

- 1 tablespoon olive oil
- 15 oz can of chickpeas
- 1 teaspoon kosher salt
- 1 teaspoon fresh rosemary (finely chopped)
- 1 teaspoon any spice of your choice

Tools required

- can opener
- paper towels or dishtowel
- strainer
- oven
- baking sheet
- measuring spoons

Procedure

1. Preheat the oven to 400 degrees with a rack placed in the center.
2. Open the can of chickpeas. Empty the contents in a strainer. Rinse the chickpeas under the running water.
3. Take one or two paper towels, or a dish towel and pat them so that they become dry.
4. Spread a layer of the chickpeas on a baking sheet that has a rim. Add some salt and olive oil. Use your hand or one spatula to mix gently so that all the chickpeas get evenly coated.
5. Roast the chickpeas in the oven for 20-30 minutes. Stir the contents or shake the pan at 10-minute intervals.
6. When they become slightly darkened and golden in color, they are ready. Their outer part will be crispy and dry while their inner portion will be soft.
7. Take them out of the oven. Sprinkle the rosemary and spices and stir or toss so that they are mixed evenly.
8. You can serve them when they are warm or keep them for later use.

Cherries on Celery Sticks

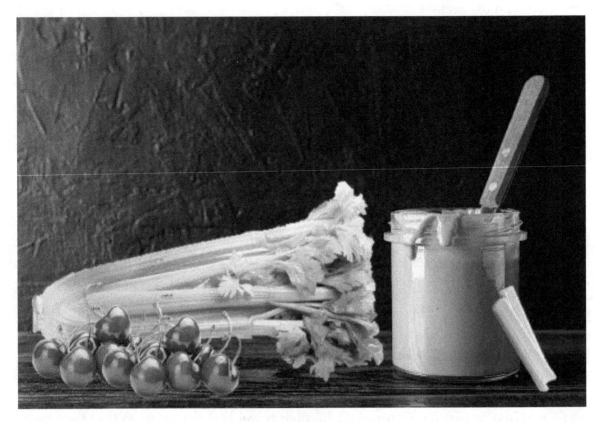

These tasty bite-sized sticks will become your favorite snack when you're feeling hungry. Celery sticks contain very few calories. For example, a cup of celery is only 16 calories. Therefore, it can help in maintaining a healthy weight and controlling diabetes.

Besides this, it contains antioxidants known as flavonoids, which play a significant role in bringing down blood sugar levels.

Time: 5 minutes

Serves: 1

Nutritional Facts: 96 Calories | 8.1 g Fats | 3.7 g Carbs | 4.1 g Protein

Ingredients

- 1 tbsp peanut butter (natural)
- 2 celery sticks (4 inches each)
- 4 cherries

Procedure

1. Wash the celery sticks and cherries with tap water.
2. Spread the peanut butter on the celery sticks.
3. Place them on a plate
4. Arrange the cherries on the sticks and serve.

Energy Bites

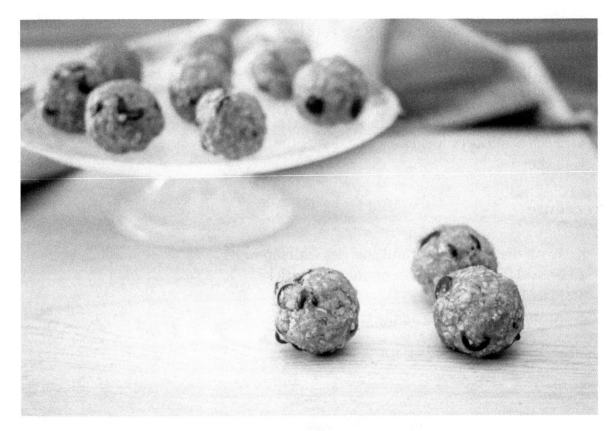

These energy bites will keep you fueled during the day. You can make them by mixing some of your favorite ingredients like oats, peanut butter, and seeds. Mostly the items used for making these bites contain plenty of healthy fats, fiber, and protein which help to stabilize the blood sugar levels.

Above all, they're easy to make, and you can take them in your bag wherever you go.

Time: 30 minutes

Serves: 20

Nutritional Facts: 130 Calories | 7 g Fats | 14 g Carbs | 3 g Protein

Ingredients

- 1 teaspoon vanilla extract
- 4 oz peanut butter
- 2.5 oz honey
- 8 oz oats (rolled)
- 5 oz shredded coconut (toasted, sweetened)
- 4 oz flaxseed meal (golden)
- 3 oz chocolate chips

Procedure

1. Put the peanut butter, vanilla extract, and honey in a bowl and mix them together.
2. Add in the rest of the ingredients. Stir until they are mixed evenly.
3. Transfer the mixture to a freezer or refrigerator. Chill the mixture for 25 minutes so that it becomes firm.
4. Take the mixture out from the fridge and make small balls around 1-inch in size.
5. You can put the balls in a large bowl or plate and serve them. If you want to save them for later, you can put them in one airtight container and store them in the fridge.

Note:

- You can use unsweetened coconut instead of the sweetened variety. Remember to purchase shredded coconut. Do not buy coconut flakes (Jaclyn, 2014).

Blueberry and Lemon Smoothie

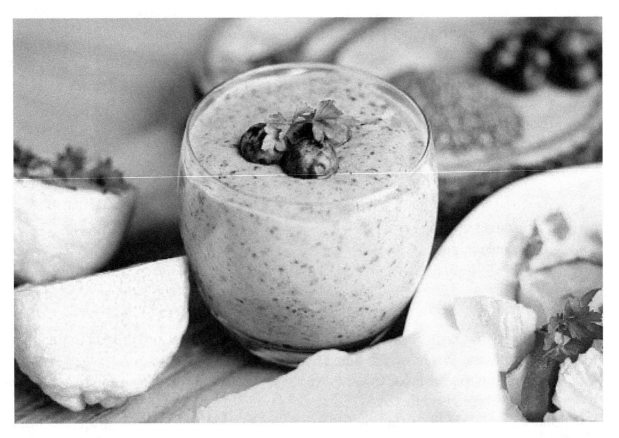

This tasty, nutritious smoothie makes a perfect breakfast or snack. The citrus fruits provide vitamin C, potassium, and folate without the added carbs. The blueberries also have plenty of fiber and antioxidants so that you can gain a lot of health benefits in one drink.

Time: 5 minutes

Serves: 1

Nutritional Facts: 293 Calories | 21.1 g Fats | 27.4 g Carbs | 3.8 g Protein

Ingredients

- 1 oz frozen blueberries
- 1/2 banana
- 1/4 oz oats (rolled)
- 1/8 tablespoons lemon zest
- 1 teaspoon lemon juice
- 3 oz almond milk (unsweetened)

Procedure

1. Put all the items in a blender. Blend for about 30 seconds to 1 minute until a smooth mixture is formed. Pour the contents in a glass and enjoy.

Pineapple and Mango Smoothie

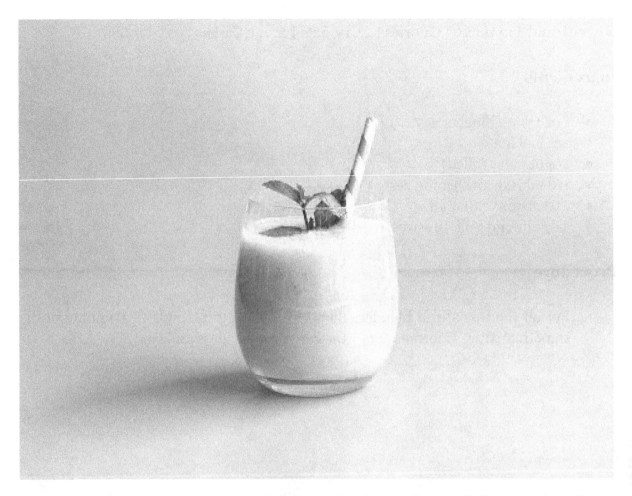

Mangoes are good for people with diabetes. They have plenty of fiber, so they do not increase the levels of blood sugar as much as other fruits, like papayas which have less fiber. Besides this, they contain fructose. This is a kind of sugar brings about very little change in the blood sugar levels compared to the other types of sugar, such as sucrose and glucose.

However, pineapple, which is one of the main ingredients, has a high-GI and may increase blood sugar levels if consumed in larger quantities. Therefore, you should not have more than one serving at a time.

Lastly, this recipe contains chia seeds which have plenty of fiber and less digestible carbs. You already know that fiber slows down the movement of food through the gut as well as its absorption, which prevents the blood glucose levels from rising.

Time: 5 minutes

Serves: 1

Nutritional Facts: 349 Calories | 29.1 g Fats | 20.6 g Carbs | 6.8 g Protein

Ingredients

- 1/2 oz pineapple slices (frozen)
- 1/2 oz mango slices (frozen)
- 1/2 oz chia seeds
- 3 oz almond milk (unsweetened)

Procedure

1. Put all the ingredients in a blender. Blend for around 30 seconds or 1 minute until a smooth mixture is formed. Then pour the contents in a glass and enjoy.

Note:

It is convenient to use frozen fruits since they give a nice texture to the smoothies. However, you can use fresh fruits instead. When using the fresh varieties, you can add a few ice cubes before blending. Besides this, you can add any extras to the smoothies according to your choice.

In the next chapter, I've provided a 14-day meal plan using the recipes mentioned.

Chapter 12: 14-Day Diabetes Meal Plan

This 14-day meal plan includes recipes for breakfast, lunch, snacks, and dinner. You can see the nutritional value of each recipe below. The nutritional value of all the recipes included each day are added up and given as the nutritional value for the day. Similarly, the nutritional values for seven days have been totaled to calculate the nutritional value for a week. However, feel free to experiment and customized your meal plan according to your personal needs and tastes.

Day 1

- **Breakfast:** Turkey Rolls
  Nutritional Facts: 155 Calories | 4.5 g Fats | 7.5 g Carbs | 22.9 g Protein
- **Lunch:** Roasted Beet, Pear and Walnut Salad
  Nutritional Facts: 438 Calories | 28.2 g Fats | 34.9 g Carbs | 16.2 g Protein
- **Snacks:** Yogurt and Berries
  Nutritional Facts: 216 Calories | 3.3 g Fats | 27.8 g Carbs | 14.5 g Protein
- **Dinner:** Arctic Char Soup
  Nutritional Facts: 535 Calories | 30.9 g Fats | 15.1 g Carbs | 8.4 g Protein

Total Nutritional Value for the Day:

Nutritional Facts: 1344 Calories | 66.9 g Fats | 85.3 g Carbs | 62 g Protein

Day 2

- **Breakfast:** Low Carb Egg Bowl
  Nutritional Facts: 178 Calories | 14.3 g Fats | 7.6 g Carbs | 6.9 g Protein
- **Lunch:** Chicken Salad with Ginger and Sesame Dressing
  Nutritional Facts: 71 Calories | 1.1 g Fats | 9.6 g Carbs | 6.6 g Protein
- **Snacks:** Peanut Butter and Apple
  Nutritional Facts: 105 Calories | 4.2 g Fats | 17 g Carbs | 2.3 g Protein
- **Dinner:** Turkey, Cauliflower and Kale Soup
  Nutritional Facts: 356 Calories | 13.3 g Fats | 21.7 g Carbs | 39 g Protein

Total Nutritional Value for the Day:

Nutritional Facts: 710 Calories | 32.9 g Fats | 55.9 g Carbs | 54.8 g Protein

Day 3

- **Breakfast:** Tasty Wrap
  Nutritional Facts: 362 Calories | 19.5 g Fats | 27 g Carbs | 23.1 g Protein
- **Lunch:** Tuna Salad Mediterranean Style
  Nutritional Facts: 183 Calories | 6.1 g Fats | 22.5 g Carbs | 10.9 g Protein
- **Snacks:** Roasted Chickpeas
  Nutritional Facts: 89.5 Calories | 3.2 g Fats | 12.2 g Carbs | 3.7 g Protein
- **Dinner:** Healthy Escarole and Chicken Soup
  Nutritional Facts: 542 Calories | 22.6 g Fats | 23.5 g Carbs | 60.9 g Protein

Total Nutritional Value for the Day:

Nutritional Facts: 1176.5 Calories | 51.4 g Fats | 85.2 g Carbs | 98.6 g Protein

Day 4

- **Breakfast:** Carrot Hummus
  Nutritional Facts: 168 Calories | 9 g Fats | 19.2 g Carbs | 4.5 g Protein
- **Lunch:** Chicken Meatballs
  Nutritional Facts: 549 Calories | 30.6 g Fats | 24.2 g Carbs | 39.8 g Protein
- **Snacks:** Cherries on Celery Sticks
  Nutritional Facts: 96 Calories | 8.1 g Fats | 3.7 g Carbs | 4.1 g Protein
- **Dinner:** Nachos Healthy Soup
  Nutritional Facts: 339 Calories | 20.7 g Fats | 26.9 g Carbs | 16.4 g Protein

Total Nutritional Value for the Day:

Nutritional Facts: 1152 Calories | 68.4 g Fats | 74 g Carbs | 64.8 g Protein

Day: 5

- **Breakfast:** Avocado Toast
  Nutritional Facts: 339 Calories | 27.9 g Fats | 15.2 g Carbs | 9.7 g Protein
- **Lunch:** Teriyaki-Braised Greens and Turnips with Bacon
  Nutritional Facts: 187 Calories | 4.3 g Fats | 29.4 g Carbs | 8.1 g Protein
- **Snacks:** Energy Bites
  Nutritional Facts: 130 Calories | 7 g Fats | 14 g Carbs | 3 g Protein
- **Dinner:** Sweet Potato and Harissa Soup
  Nutritional Facts: 215 Calories | 11.5 g Fats | 22.5 g Carbs | 7.8 g Protein

Total Nutritional Value for the Day:

Nutritional Facts: 871 Calories | 50.7 g Fats | 81.1 g Carbs | 28.6 g Protein

Day 6

- **Breakfast:** Chia Pudding
  Nutritional Facts: 155 Calories | 8 g Fats | 16 g Carbs | 4 g Protein
- **Lunch:** Broccoli and Barley Risotto with Basil and Lemon
  Nutritional Facts: 195 Calories | 7.6 g Fats | 28.9 g Carbs | 4.5 g Protein
- **Snacks:** Blueberry and Lemon Smoothie
  Nutritional Facts: 293 Calories | 21.1 g Fats | 27.4 g Carbs | 3.8 g Protein
- **Dinner:** Pumpkin and Lentil Soup
  Nutritional Facts: 128 Calories | 1 g Fats | 20.8 g Carbs | 9.2 g Protein

Total Nutritional Value for the Day:

Nutritional Facts: 771 Calories | 37.7 g Fats | 93.1 g Carbs | 21.5 g Protein

Day 7

- **Breakfast:** Paleo Carrot and Pumpkin Muffins
  Nutritional Facts: 185 Calories | 11 g Fats | 19 g Carbs | 6 g Protein
- **Lunch:** Blueberry and Avocado Salsa
  Nutritional Facts: 137 Calories | 10 g Fats | 12.5 g Carbs | 1.7 g Protein
- **Snacks:** Pineapple and Mango Smoothie
  Nutritional Facts: 349 Calories | 29.1 g Fats | 20.6 g Carbs | 6.8 g Protein
- **Dinner:** Sprouted Lentils with Vegan Stew
  Nutritional Facts: 211 Calories | 7.6 g Fats | 27.1 g Carbs | 10.1 g Protein

Total Nutritional Value for the Day:

Nutritional Facts: 882 Calories | 57.7 g Fats | 79.2 g Carbs | 24.6 g Protein

Total Nutritional Value for the Week:

6906.5 Calories | 365.7 g Fats | 553.8 g Carbs | 354.9 g Protein

Day 8

- **Breakfast:** Turkey Rolls
  Nutritional Facts: 155 Calories | 4.5 g Fats | 7.5 g Carbs | 22.9 g Protein
- **Lunch:** Arctic Char Soup
  Nutritional Facts: 535 Calories | 30.9 g Fats | 15.1 g Carbs | 8.4 g Protein
- **Snacks:** Yogurt and Berries
  Nutritional Facts: 216 Calories | 3.3 g Fats | 27.8 g Carbs | 14.5 g Protein
- **Dinner:** Roasted Beet, Pear and Walnut Salad
  Nutritional Facts: 438 Calories | 28.2 g Fats | 34.9 g Carbs | 16.2 g Protein

Total Nutritional Value for the Day:

Nutritional Facts: 1344 Calories | 66.9 g Fats | 85.3 g Carbs | 62 g Protein

Day 9

- **Breakfast:** Low Carb Egg Bowl
  Nutritional Facts: 178 Calories | 14.3 g Fats | 7.6 g Carbs | 6.9 g Protein
- **Lunch:** Turkey, Cauliflower and Kale Soup
  Nutritional Facts: 356 Calories | 13.3 g Fats | 21.7 g Carbs | 39 g Protein
- **Snacks:** Peanut Butter and Apple
  Nutritional Facts: 105 Calories | 4.2 g Fats | 17 g Carbs | 2.3 g Protein
- **Dinner:** Chicken Salad with Ginger and Sesame Dressing
  Nutritional Facts: 71 Calories | 1.1 g Fats | 9.6 g Carbs | 6.6 g Protein

Total Nutritional Value for the Day:

Nutritional Facts: 710 Calories | 32.9 g Fats | 55.9 g Carbs | 54.8 g Protein

Day 10

- **Breakfast:** Tasty Wrap
  Nutritional Facts: 362 Calories | 19.5 g Fats | 27 g Carbs | 23.1 g Protein
- **Lunch:** Healthy Escarole and Chicken Soup
  Nutritional Facts: 542 Calories | 22.6 g Fats | 23.5 g Carbs | 60.9 g Protein
- **Snacks:** Roasted Chickpeas
  Nutritional Facts: 89.5 Calories | 3.2 g Fats | 12.2 g Carbs | 3.7 g Protein
- **Dinner:** Tuna Salad Mediterranean Style
  Nutritional Facts: 183 Calories | 6.1 g Fats | 22.5 g Carbs | 10.9 g Protein

Total Nutritional Value for the Day:

Nutritional Facts: 1176.5 Calories | 51.4 g Fats | 85.2 g Carbs | 98.6 g Protein

Day 11

- **Breakfast:** Carrot Hummus
  Nutritional Facts: 168 Calories | 9 g Fats | 19.2 g Carbs | 4.5 g Protein
- **Lunch:** Nachos Healthy Soup
  Nutritional Facts: 339 Calories | 20.7 g Fats | 26.9 g Carbs | 16.4 g Protein
- **Snacks:** Cherries on Celery Sticks
  Nutritional Facts: 96 Calories | 8.1 g Fats | 3.7 g Carbs | 4.1 g Protein
- **Dinner:** Chicken Meatballs
  Nutritional Facts: 549 Calories | 30.6 g Fats | 24.2 g Carbs | 39.8 g Protein

Total Nutritional Value for the Day:

Nutritional Facts: 1152 Calories | 68.4 g Fats | 74 g Carbs | 64.8 g Protein

Day 12

- **Breakfast:** Avocado Toast
  Nutritional Facts: 339 Calories | 27.9 g Fats | 15.2 g Carbs | 9.7 g Protein
- **Lunch:** Sweet Potato and Harissa Soup
  Nutritional Facts: 215 Calories | 11.5 g Fats | 22.5 g Carbs | 7.8 g Protein
- **Snacks:** Energy Bites
  Nutritional Facts: 130 Calories | 7 g Fats | 14 g Carbs | 3 g Protein
- **Dinner:** Teriyaki-Braised Greens and Turnips with Bacon
  Nutritional Facts: 187 Calories | 4.3 g Fats | 29.4 g Carbs | 8.1 g Protein

Total Nutritional Value for the Day:

Nutritional Facts: 871 Calories | 50.7 g Fats | 81.1 g Carbs | 28.6 g Protein

Day 13

- **Breakfast:** Chia Pudding
  Nutritional Facts: 155 Calories | 8 g Fats | 16 g Carbs | 4 g Protein
- **Lunch:** Pumpkin and Lentil Soup
  Nutritional Facts: 128 Calories | 1 g Fats | 20.8 g Carbs | 9.2 g Protein
- **Snacks:** Blueberry and Lemon Smoothie
  Nutritional Facts: 293 Calories | 21.1 g Fats | 27.4 g Carbs | 3.8 g Protein
- **Dinner:** Broccoli and Barley Risotto with Basil and Lemon
  Nutritional Facts: 195 Calories | 7.6 g Fats | 28.9 g Carbs | 4.5 g Protein

Total Nutritional Value for the Day:

Nutritional Facts: 771 Calories | 37.7 g Fats | 93.1 g Carbs | 21.5 g Protein

Day 14

- **Breakfast:** Paleo Carrot and Pumpkin Muffins
  Nutritional Facts: 185 Calories | 11 g Fats | 19 g Carbs | 6 g Protein
- **Lunch:** Sprouted Lentils with Vegan Stew
  Nutritional Facts: 211 Calories | 7.6 g Fats | 27.1 g Carbs | 10.1 g Protein
- **Snacks:** Pineapple and Mango Smoothie
  Nutritional Facts: 349 Calories | 29.1 g Fats | 20.6 g Carbs | 6.8 g Protein
- **Dinner:** Blueberry and Avocado Salsa
  Nutritional Facts: 137 Calories | 10 g Fats | 12.5 g Carbs | 1.7 g Protein

Total Nutritional Value for the Day:

Nutritional Facts: 882 Calories | 57.7 g Fats | 79.2 g Carbs | 24.6 g Protein

Total Nutritional Value for the Week:

6906.5 Calories | 365.7 g Fats | 553.8 g Carbs | 354.9 g Protein

Final Thoughts

We have finally reached the end of this book. I hope it has helped you to have a better understanding of this condition. We have learned a lot, including the causes, symptoms, and treatment of diabetes. You have also seen that it can be avoided and even reversed by changing your diet and lifestyle.

Thomas Edison's quote, "The doctor of the future will give no medicine but will involve the patient in the proper use of food, fresh air and exercise," (Villanueva, 2014) is quite relevant in this context.

So, you may still be wondering what you should do next?

Here are some steps to take to help prevent diabetes or to manage the symptoms of the disease:

Step 1: Follow the diabetes diet plan

According to the American Diabetes Association, the main things to be kept in mind while following a diet that is beneficial for those with diabetes are:

- Include vegetables and fruits.
- Consume lean protein.
- Avoid foods with added sugar.
- Stay away from trans fats.

To summarize, you should consume more healthy fats derived from avocados, nuts, flax seeds, fish oils, and olive oil. Eat plenty of vegetables and fruits, especially the fresh and colorful ones. Also, try to eat more whole fruits instead of drinking juices.

Make it a point to include whole-grain bread and cereals, organic turkey or chicken, shellfish, and fish in your meals. Remember to add high-quality proteins like unsweetened yogurt, dairy products that have low-fat, beans, and eggs in your daily menu.

Be careful about the number of trans fats that are found in deep-fried or partially hydrogenated foods and cut down on their consumption. Avoid processed red meat, fast food, and packaged food items, especially those that have a high sugar content like sweets and desserts.

Minimize the consumption of sugary cereals, white bread, and refined rice or pasta. Stay away from low-fat food products which have added sugars instead of fats.

Eat at fixed times because if you eat at regular intervals, your body can regulate your weight and blood glucose levels better. Start the day with a healthy breakfast so that you get sufficient energy and your blood glucose levels don't go beyond 140 mg/dL after two hours of eating.

You can eat small meals six times every day. So, the size of the servings at each meal will not be very large. Instead of eating too much in one meal or day and then skipping meals the next day, it's better to consume the same amount of food every day.

Maintain a food journal or diary. According to a study that was conducted recently, people who keep a record of their food can lose double the amount of weight compared to those who do not do so (Segal, Robinson & Smith, 2019).

The reason for this is that when you write things down, it becomes easier to identify the problem areas. For instance, when you refer to your diary, you may find that you are getting too many calories from your morning latte or afternoon snacks. This helps you to take appropriate action to cut down the calories. Keeping a journal also makes you more aware of what you are eating and the amount that you are consuming.

If you're having trouble about what foods to eat, you can refer to chapter 5 for the foods to eat on a diabetes diet. The recipes and meal plan will also help you to get started to eating better to improve your condition.

Step 2: Become more active

You can improve your body's sensitivity to insulin and also avoid gaining weight by doing exercises. Start by walking for 20 minutes, three times a week. Gradually, you can take up other exercises and engage in activities like biking and swimming. You can refer to chapter 3 for exercise tips and ideas.

Some studies have shown that intermittent fasting may be beneficial for insulin and blood glucose levels. However, further research has to be done. If you are planning to do intermittent fasting, be sure to talk to your doctor and be sure that it is safe for you to do so since fasting for low periods of time can impact your blood glucose levels.

By improving your diet and lifestyle, this will help you improve your health and hopefully avoid developing or worsening diabetes. And if you already have some the symptoms, these steps will enable you to manage them more efficiently.

I wish you all the best on your journey to a better, healthier life.

Review Request

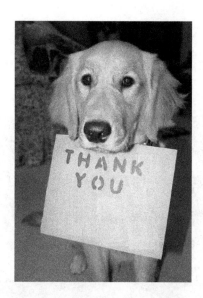

If you enjoyed this book or found it useful, then I'd like to ask you for a quick favor: would you be kind enough to leave a review for this book? It'd be greatly appreciated.

Your feedback does matter and helps me to make improvements so I can provide the best content possible.

Thank you!

Further reading

The 20-Minute Mediterranean Diet Cookbook:

Quick and Delicious Mediterranean Recipes for Weight Loss and Health

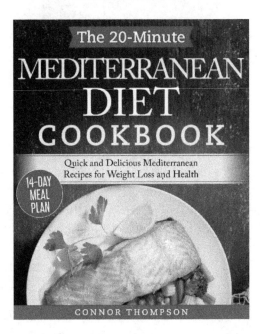

Most of us are aware of the Mediterranean diet and why it is one of the healthiest diets in the world. Millions of people now follow its principles of lots of lean meat and fresh vegetables, oily fish and succulent fruit, and it has gained popularity around the globe with some truly outstanding and memorable dishes.

Now, in **The 20-Minute Mediterranean Diet Cookbook,** you can recreate the taste of the Mediterranean faster than ever before, and all in the comfort of your own kitchen, with information on:

- **Health benefits of the Mediterranean diet and the diseases it can help combat**
- **The types of food to eat and those to avoid**
- **Meal prepping and its benefits for you**

- **Shopping lists for an easy life**
- **Tips for success and FAQs**
- **A 14-day meal plan**
- **Lots of tasty recipes for you to try**
- **And lots more...**

Of course, it isn't just the speed of these recipes that is the great feature of this book, with recipes taking just **20 minutes** to make, you also get lots of information on the history and benefits of the diet, top tips for success and a 14-day meal plan to get you started.

If you ever thought that the Mediterranean diet could be for you, start now, with **The 20-Minute Mediterranean Diet Cookbook!**

http://bit.ly/20min-mediterranean-diet

The Science of Intermittent Fasting:

The Complete Guide to Unlocking Your Weight Loss Potential

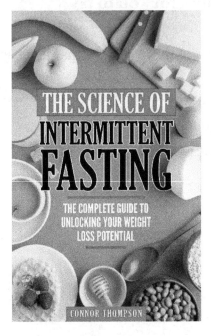

Are you thinking about losing weight or have you been trying to lose weight unsuccessfully?

Are you ready to try something that will shed those excess pounds and boost your heath?

In, *The Science of Intermittent Fasting,* you can discover how intermittent fasting could work for you, through chapters that look at:

- **What intermittent fasting is all about**
- **Cellular repair**
- **Improving brain health**
- **Optimizing your insulin, leptin and ghrelin levels**
- **Inflammation**
- **Cholesterol**
- **Cancer and diabetes**
- **Aging**
- **How to get the most out of your fasts**
- **And lots more...**

The scientific benefits of intermittent fasting on your health and weight loss are clear to see and with an in-depth look into the research and studies carried out on intermittent fasting, ***The Science of Intermittent Fasting*** is the perfect book that deliver all the answers.

Get a copy today and see for yourself how intermittent fasting can not only be good for your weight, but good for your whole body.

http://bit.ly/thescienceoffastingbook

References

Avocado Toast. Retrieved from
https://www.ninjakitchen.com/recipes/search/0/all/101478/avocado-toast/

BBC Good Food team. (2016, June). Barley & broccoli risotto with lemon & basil. Retrieved from https://www.bbcgoodfood.com/recipes/barley-broccoli-risotto-lemon-basil

Brain booster wrap. (2008, January 1). Retrieved fromhttps://www.food24.com/Recipes/Brain-booster-wrap-20091103-2

Caceres, V. (2017, April 11). What Are the Causes of Diabetes? Retrieved from https://health.usnews.com/health-care/patient-advice/articles/2017-04-11/what-are-the-causes-of-diabetes

California Avocado Red, White and Blueberry Salsa. Retrieved from

https://www.californiaavocado.com/recipe-details/view/31618/california-avocado-red-white-and-blueberry-salsa

Carrot Hummus. Retrieved from
https://www.ninjakitchen.com/recipes/search/0/all/101726/carrot-hummus/ Chicken sage tagliatelle. Retrieved from

https://www.food24.com/Recipes-and-Menus/Easy-Weekday-Meals/chicken-sage-tagliatelle-20151116-2

Christensen, E. (updated 2019, December 20). How to make crispy roasted chickpeas in the oven. Retrieved from https://www.thekitchn.com/how-to-make-crispy-roasted-chickpeas-in-the-oven-cooking-lessons-from-the-kitchn-219753

Cleveland Clinic Health Essentials team. (2015, October 31). Pumpkin Lentil Soup. Retrieved from https://healthybrains.org/pumpkin-lentil-soup/

Cleveland Clinic Wellness. (2017, February 10). Brain Healthy Chicken and Escarole. Retrieved from https://healthybrains.org/soups-brain-healthy-chicken-escarole/

Donofrio, J. (n.d.). Roasted Beet Salad with Pear and Walnuts. Retrieved fromhttps://www.loveandlemons.com/roasted-beet-salad/

Donovan, J. (n.d.). Weight and Diabetes: Lose Pounds to Lower Your Risk. Retrieved from https://www.webmd.com/diabetes/features/diabetes-weight-loss-finding-the-right-path#1

Elliott, B. (2018, January 14). The 21 best snack ideas if you have diabetes. Retrieved from https://www.healthline.com/nutrition/best-snacks-for-diabetes

Izzy. (2019, June 24). Healthy smoothie recipes - 6 flavors. Retrieved from https://www.shelikesfood.com/healthy-smoothie-recipes/

Jaclyn. (2014, April 28). No bake energy bites. Retrieved from https://www.cookingclassy.com/no-bake-energy-bites/

Jawad, Y. (2018, June 23). 3 Ingredient chia pudding. Retrieved from https://feelgoodfoodie.net/recipe/3-ingredient-chia-pudding/

Killeen, B. (2018, March/April). Fire Ants on a Log. Retrieved from http://www.eatingwell.com/recipe/262760/fire-ants-on-a-log/

Killeen, B. (2018, March/April). Roasted Salmon with Smoky Chickpeas & Greens. Retrieved from http://www.eatingwell.com/recipe/262763/roasted-salmon-with-smoky-chickpeas-greens/

McDermott, A. and Gotter, A. (2016, May 10). 10 Diabetes diet myths. Retrieved from https://www.healthline.com/health/diabetes/diet-myths#sugar-and-diabetes

Mediterranean tuna salad. Retrieved from https://www.food24.com/Recipes/mediterranean-tuna-salad-2017031

Mullins, B. (2015, November 16). Hard Boiled Egg and Avocado Bowl. Retrieved from https://www.eatingbirdfood.com/hardboiled-egg-and-avocado-bowl/#tasty-recipes-33961 Nachos soup. Retrieved from https://www.food24.com/Perfect-Balance/nachos-soup-20190530

Nelson, B. (2014, November). Teriyaki-Braised Turnips and Greens with Bacon. Retrieved from https://experiencelife.com/recipe/teriyaki-braised-turnips-and-greens-with-bacon/

Nguyen, N.T. and others. (2010, December 3). Relationship Between Obesity and Diabetes in a US Adult Population: Findings from the National Health and Nutrition Examination Survey, 1999–2006. Retrieved from https://www.ncbi.nlm.nih.gov/pmc/articles/PMC3040808/

Nunavut Development Corporation. (n.d.). Arctic Char Chowder. Retrieved fromhttp://www.trulywild.ca/Recipes/Arctic%20Char%20Chowder

Oberg, E. (n.d.). Type 2diabetes diet plan. Retrieved from https://www.medicinenet.com/diabetic_diet_for_type_2_diabetes/article.htm

Overhiser, S. & A. (n.d.). Vegan Stew with Sprouted Lentils. Retrieved fromhttps://www.acouplecooks.com/hearty-sprouted-lentil-stew-with-kale/

Overhiser, S. & A. (n.d.). Vegan Sweet Potato Soup with Harissa. Retrieved fromhttps://www.acouplecooks.com/sweet-potato-soup-harissa-greens/

Pietrangelo, A. (2019, May 28). Understanding type 2 diabetes. Retrieved from https://www.healthline.com/health/type-2-diabetes

Quotes from diabetics - Lifestyle of a type 2 diabetes patient. Retrieved from https://sites.google.com/site/lifestyleoftype2/quotes-from-diabetics

Roland, J. (2017, June 29). Signs of insulin resistance. Retrieved from https://www.healthline.com/health/diabetes/insulin-resistance-symptoms

Schaeffer, J. (2018, June 27). Understanding borderline diabetes: Signs, symptoms, and more. Retrieved from https://www.healthline.com/health/diabetes/borderline-diabetes-know-the-signs

Segal, J., Robinson, L., and Smith, M. (updated 2019, November). The diabetes diet. Retrieved from https://www.helpguide.org/articles/diets/the-diabetes-diet.htm

Sissons, B. (2019, February 12). What are the best foods for people with diabetes? Retrieved from https://www.medicalnewstoday.com/articles/324416.php

Spritzler, F. (2017, June 3). The 16 best foods to control diabetes. Retrieved from https://www.healthline.com/nutrition/16-best-foods-for-diabetics

Tam, M. (n.d.). Paleo Pumpkin and Carrot Muffins. Retrieved from https://nomnompaleo.com/post/101828602863/paleo-pumpkin-and-carrot-muffins

Tello, M. (2018, September 6). Healthy lifestyle can prevent diabetes (and even reverse it). Retrieved from https://www.health.harvard.edu/blog/healthy-lifestyle-can-prevent-diabetes-and-even-reverse-it-2018090514698

Townley, C. (2018, October 13). Intermittent fasting may help fight type 2 diabetes. Retrieved from https://www.medicalnewstoday.com/articles/323316.php

Turkey, Kale, and Cauliflower Soup. Retrieved from https://paleoleap.com/turkey-kale-cauliflower-soup/

Villanueva, B. (2014, April 4). 12 Motivational quotes for diabetics. Retrieved from https://tgp.com.ph/blog/12-motivational-quotes-diabetes/

Williams, B. (n.d.). The Ratio of Fats, Carbohydrates & Protein for Diabetics. Retrieved from https://www.livestrong.com/article/363268-the-ratio-of-fats-carbohydrates-protein-for-diabetics/

CPSIA information can be obtained
at www.ICGtesting.com
Printed in the USA
LVHW100805010221
677982LV00011B/375